Challenges in Caring

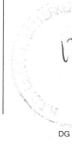

Challenges in Caring

Explorations in nursing and ethics

JAMES M. BROWN

*Senior Lecturer in Philosophy,
University of Ulster at Coleraine,
Northern Ireland*

ALISON L. KITSON

*Director,
The Royal College of Nursing 'Standards of Care'
Project and Head of Research and Evaluation,
Institute of Nursing
Oxford*

and

TERENCE J. MCKNIGHT

*Lecturer in Philosophy,
University of Ulster at Coleraine,
Northern Ireland*

Stanley Thornes (Publishers) Ltd

First edition published by Chapman & Hall in 1992 (ISBN 0–412–34400–9)

Reprinted in 1997 by:
Stanley Thornes (Publishers) Ltd
Ellenborough House
Wellington Street
CHELTENHAM
GL50 1YW
United Kingdom

97 98 99 00 01 / 10 9 8 7 6 5 4 3 2 1

A catalogue record for this book is available from the British Library.

ISBN 0–7487–3283–7

Typeset by Intype, London
Printed and bound in Great Britain by Athenaeum Press, Gateshead

Contents

Preface

Changes in biomedical technology, in institutional health care, in nursing, and in society increasingly cause nurses to be in situations requiring them to take moral decisions or to be involved in the consequences of such decisions. For the sake of patients, good practice, personal integrity and self-respect, nurses need to be able to satisfy themselves and sometimes others that their particular decisions and general practices are defensible. The aim of this book is to assist those in the nursing profession who seek to cope clear-headedly and responsibly with moral issues; it should leave the reader better placed to articulate the moral considerations and underlying principles bearing upon such issues – even if they do not agree with the present authors about what these are.

This book is concerned with problems and situations of a kind that are central to nursing. It is addressed to everyone who has moral concerns with such problems and situations. Suppose we were to set out certain fundamental principles of our own and then just apply those principles to those problems and situations. We should then in effect just be speaking to people who already shared those fundamental principles. There would be no reason why anyone else should pay any attention to us. Indeed if morality could only be the application of a fixed set of fundamental principles to situations and problems, then there would be no reason for anyone to pay attention to what people with different first principles had to say about moral matters.

But moral thinking cannot be just the application of principles to problems and situations. Most people do not even know what their principles are, and we, writing this book, would be extremely hard pressed to give a definitive statement of our fundamental principles. We could of course try to articulate some principles, and no doubt we should come up with some plausible ones. But we could not be certain that the implications of those principles would always be morally acceptable to us. Any principles worth their salt would have lots of consequences which would not be apparent at first. Might not some of these non-obvious consequences be so foreign to our moral responses that we simply could not go along with them? This is a possibility that cannot be ruled out. And, if we were to find out that the principles we thought of had consequences that were morally unacceptable to us, we should have to change the principles. In a sense, moral discussion sincerely entered into is as much a process of discovering one's principles as it is a process of applying principles.

In addressing ourselves to all those who are concerned with the situations and problems that we are concerned with, we are trying to contribute to a continuing process of moral discovery. Moral discussion among people with shared moral concerns is always potentially fruitful: we may make progress towards moral consensus on solutions to outstanding moral problems, and even where we do not move towards consensus we do learn more about our own principles.

The book is in part a response to an expressed need within the profession for more critical thinking. Instead of letting moral thinking be guided largely by unspoken assumptions, the book tries to get the reader into the habit of articulating such assumptions – their own and other people's – and, where appropriate, subjecting them to critical examination.

The book will put the reader in a position to identify and analyse recurring moral issues which are characteristic of nursing practice; and it will acquaint them with the standard arguments relating to those issues. However, it aspires to do much more than that. In situations which previously would just have left a diffuse sense of frustration or an uneasy feeling that somewhere something is not quite right, we hope that the reader of this book will afterwards be able much more swiftly and confidently to put their finger on just what it is about the situation that is questionable and just why it evokes disquiet.

We intend the book to be suitable for use in courses on ethics in nursing. For lectures corresponding to some parts of the book there are overhead projector transparencies, prepared on an Apple Macintosh computer using HyperCard. If any reader wants to see what they look like please write to James Brown in the Department of Philosophy and Politics, The University of Ulster at Coleraine. Anyone who wants the files to use should send a Macintosh disk which will then be returned with the files. In general, we would be eager to hear from anyone who is engaged in ethics courses for nurses.

We have several debts of gratitude to be recorded. The immensity of what we have learned from students of the University of Ulster – and before that the New University of Ulster – makes us wonder who is meant to be teaching whom. A lot of collaborative work for this book has been done at a distance, but we are grateful to the Faculty of Humanities in the University of Ulster for enabling us to work together in Oxford for a very fruitful week, and to the Institute of Nursing for hospitably providing space and a friendly atmosphere. We benefited from the boundless patience, understanding, and support of Christine Birdsall who took us and our project on, and of Rosemary Morris who saw it through to the end. We have learned a great deal from conversations with Pat Ashworth, who also kindly read parts of the draft manuscript. Peter Brown read an early draft of several chapters and made useful comments on them.

As well as those debts that we have incurred as a team, we each have personal acknowledgements to make. Over many years Marlis Prem and Peter Brown have told James Brown far more about their experiences and concerns in nursing than he can say. And, rather for helping to shape a life than for support with this particular project, he also wishes to thank parents, spouse, and children, and the philosophers Dorothy Emmet and Nicholas Maxwell. For his part, Terry McKnight would like to thank all the nurses with whom he has discussed ethical dilemmas over the years and hopes that after all this time he is as sensitive to the real problems as they would wish, and, in particular, he would like to thank his family for their patience and fortitude during the work on this project and over the years. Alison Kitson would also like to acknowledge the help and support received from both nursing colleagues and friends in the philosophy department at the University of Ulster and elsewhere. Without the searching questions of the philosophers, the insight and experience of the clinicians can often evaporate away. Thanks also to family and friends, especially 'my boys' for their patience and support.

James M. Brown
Alison L. Kitson
Terence J. McKnight

ONE

Moral thinking

1.1 A MORAL PROBLEM

'Am I going to die, nurse?'

The patient wants an answer from you. You know he is dying. A quick decision and response is needed.

Perhaps you have been in this situation. Was it easy to see what to do? Did you feel afterwards that you chose the right option? Did you feel that there might be another option which had not even occurred to you?

Many nurses find this a troubling situation. They cope with it, in one way or another. But they often continue to feel uneasy. Their unease is not about the legality of the response. It is not just about whether the UKCC code of conduct was followed. It is not just about whether the response is the one the doctor would have insisted on. The unease is about whether the response was the right one, the best available response for all concerned. When it is put like this, the nature of the unease is left pretty vague. But that is reasonable. Moral reflection starts from a sense that some things are rather important and worth worrying about. People who have this sense often are not in a position to say clearly what those things are and in what ways they are important and why they are worth worrying about. What is distinctive of moral unease is something that the reader will be in a better position to say at the end of the book. For the moment, then, let us simply say that moral unease is no stranger to most nurses.

Thinking and talking about the troubling situation has a practical purpose: it leaves you less unprepared, less likely to be caught off-balance, when a similar situation arises another time.

1.2 YOU DECIDE

A nurse, like anyone else, makes her own moral decisions. No one else can make them for her. She may seek advice from someone; but it is she who decides whom to listen to and whether to act on the advice. She may have a code of conduct covering the case in hand, but it remains her decision whether to do what the code says or to disregard it (perhaps at great personal cost). A book like this one ought to be of some practical use, but its use is not that it leaves the reader with less deciding to do. As the UKCC (1987) says, 'no exploration or elaboration by others alters the fact that the ultimate decision is that of the individual practitioner in the situation'.

There is sometimes confusion about this matter of each person having to take his or her own decisions. We need to distinguish the following questions:

- Who makes the decision?
- What makes the decision correct or incorrect?
- How are we to satisfy ourselves that the decision was correct or that it was incorrect?

The UKCC (1987) is surely right to say that a moral agent ultimately makes her own decision. Of course, being the owner of the decision does not make the decision correct. It may well be that we have to look elsewhere for an appraisal of her decision.

The correctness or incorrectness of a decision can depend on various factors, such as the rights and obligations of the people involved and the good or harm that is likely to result. The person deciding may be unaware of some of these factors, and because of this they may arrive at the wrong decision.

Satisfying ourselves that a decision was correct or that it was not correct may be much easier after the event. There may then be more time to review all the relevant factors and to consider how much weight should be given to them and to discuss various aspects of the situation with people we respect. If there is doubt about the correctness of a decision then it is best resolved by such discussion.

1.3 DECIDING CAN BE DONE WELL OR BADLY

A frequent theme in film and television comedy is the harassed man who decides badly. The situation might develop as follows. An important issue arises. Perhaps the man has an opportunity to start his own shop, a lifelong ambition; but leaving his secure job would be a risky step. A decision is needed at once. The telephone rings, the doorbell rings, a water pipe bursts, the neighbours have deafening music playing, a large bird flies in through the window and blunders about looking for the way out again; in exasperation the man seizes on one possible response to the important issue. But it is plain that he has not decided well. The chances are that the outcome will be disastrous. If everything does come out right in the end it will be because of other factors and not because his deciding was done well.

Why did he not decide well? For a start, he did not review the obvious choices in a calm way. He did not search imaginatively to see whether other possible choices could be found or made. He did not reflect on the things that would be involved in each of the possible choices, and on how important or unimportant to him each of those things was – and perhaps how important it would be to him in a few years. Maybe more is involved in deciding well. But what we have said so far suffices to make it plain that deciding is something that can be done well or badly.

Of course, in the extreme circumstances of the comedy, most people would have made a poor job of deciding. But comedy is often about the character defects of the persons depicted. The character played by Woody Allen or John Cleese has certain preoccupations, certain habits of mind, a tendency for certain feelings to get out of hand, a tendency to be distracted from important matters by relatively unimportant ones, and so on. These are some of the things that go to make him the kind of person he is. And these things make it likely that his deciding will be impaired by unfavourable conditions. Even in favourable conditions, some kinds of people are more likely to decide well than others. For example, a lecturer who can think of nothing but a cherished research project is quite likely to make poor decisions in teaching, and a person who is exclusively preoccupied with promotion opportunities is likely to make a poor choice of marriage partner. So is a person who can think of nothing but string quartets.

Deciding can be done well or badly. And some kinds of people are likely to do it better than others. Ethical deciding, too, can be done well or badly. And some kinds of people are likely to do it better than others.

1.4 MUST ETHICS BE THREATENING?

Here is one view of ethics:

Ethics is about facing up to one's responsibilities, finding out where one's duty lies and acting accordingly. It is about overcoming weakness, having no thought for one's own safety or career. It is about having standards higher than other people's standards. Miners, power workers, bank staff might go on strike, but nurses should stay at their posts no matter how bad things get. Ethics is a hard and unforgiving taskmaster, setting ever harder tasks, permitting no self-satisfaction for success and punishing failure with guilt and self-reproach.

But this sounds dreadful. Many people's working lives are difficult enough without this as well. Life it too short, there is too much to be done. One is tempted to say: 'Let the theorists get on with discussing ethics and writing their articles and books. People in the real world have work to do and no time for extras, especially unattractive extras.'

As we write this book, that is not how we see ethics. We are not urging the reader to take on board a new set of problems. We are addressing ourselves to readers who have already found themselves with moral problems or who will find themselves with moral problems and who care about solving them. People who are distressed because they are instructed to do what they consider to be wrong already have a moral problem; paying attention to moral problems is not for them an optional extra. A concern with ethics is not something that one might be asked to opt into and which one might decline to opt into.

People come to have moral problems because they have certain concerns. There are some things which they think are important, and important in a special way. One kind of concern is a concern for others who are suffering. Another is a concern to do something worthwhile in one's life. Another is a concern for justice. We can have these concerns – or others like them – without being sure how best to characterize them. Even the concerns just mentioned might be more accurately described in a different way. Part of the work of ethics is to find good ways of putting the moral concerns into words so that we can more readily think about what they involve, and not only think about it but also talk about it and exchange ideas and try to criticize and improve upon one another's ideas. (The moral concerns that a person has may develop and change. No doubt the concern to please our infant class teacher was once a major factor with many of us; no doubt other concerns in due course displaced that one.)

Whatever the best characterization of those concerns is, anyone with those concerns is sometimes going to have problems that arise because of those concerns. A person who did not have those concerns would not have those problems. This book is addressed to people who do have the concerns. And, since you have the concerns, you will want to solve the problems.

In the course of the book we try to identify the concerns and to characterize them. Our attempts to do this will sometimes involve the use of strange words. Nevertheless, we hope that with the help of examples and explanations the reader will come to find that the concerns identified are familiar ones. Much of the time we will not be telling the reader new things but will be helping the reader to acquire the vocabulary to talk and think effectively about very familiar things.

So the tone of an ethics book should not be a hectoring tone. It is not a matter of telling you to take on board problems that you may not want to take on board. It is not a matter of browbeating you into doing things that you might be disinclined to do. It is about enabling you to be more effective in acting in a way that reflects the practical concerns you have.

Ethical vocabulary – talk of duty and responsibility and virtue – is sometimes used in an unscrupulous way to damp down or divert criticism of unsatisfactory arrangements; and an emphasis on the ethical responsibilities of individuals can obscure questions about the ethical character of institutions. These tendencies can foster mistrust of attempts to promote ethical discussion. However, by promoting critical awareness of ethical concepts and arguments, a book like this one should leave the reader better placed to recognize and resist the misuse or misdirection of ethical ideas.

1.5 OBJECTIVE SCIENCE AND PERSONAL FEELINGS

Morality, it is often thought, is profoundly personal and subjective and beyond the reach of rationality. Science, on the other hand, is impersonal, objective and provable. Moral thinking is thus something utterly different from scientific rationality.

This view is mistaken. Scientific rationality is not a matter of dealing only with provables. Moral convictions and moral feelings can be reconsidered and revised in the light of reasoned argument. Scientific thinking and moral thinking, when done well, often involve exercising just the same qualities of mind. Facing up to moral issues need involve no sacrifice of scientific or intellectual integrity.

Let us enlarge on the point that science is not concerned only with provables. It has long been known that scientific enquiry has to involve not just observational data but also hypotheses (see, for example, the extract from John Stuart Mill reprinted in Brown *et al.*, 1981, pp. 97–100).

For example, people see the stars every night and the changes in their positions; and those people make various guesses about how to explain them (e.g. there is a fire out there and a moving black canopy with pinholes in it screening it from us, or there are glowing heavenly bodies fixed to invisible spheres that turn about the earth, or there are a lot of lumps of hot or cold rock hurtling about in empty space obeying a few laws of motion and exerting a gravitational pull on each other). Some of these conjectural explanations become very refined and elaborate, can explain an amazing variety of what appeared to be quite separate observational facts, and make reference to things that cannot be observed. Conjectural explanations of this kind are not just humble hypotheses but are blue-blood theories. The history of science is littered with abandoned hypotheses and theories; there is every reason to suppose that some of the ones our generation cherishes will in due course be superseded. It is the fate of most theories, including some of the best, to be superseded.

Explanatory hypotheses and theories cannot possibly be proved true. This has become increasingly plain as, in the last century or so, logicians have been able to produce standards of proof far more rigorous than in earlier times. So scientific rationality consists to a great extent in seeking, having and offering to others good reasons for accepting hypotheses which cannot be proved. (Of course, some of them may be true or, while false, may be closer to the truth than others.) Scientific rationality does not consist in accepting only what is provable.

Good hypotheses can often be experimentally tested. Favourable test outcomes do not prove a hypothesis correct but may give good reason for provisional acceptance of the hypothesis. In inviting others to accept the hypothesis, an investigator may report the results of experiments already done and invite others to duplicate those results. The investigator does not say 'Trust me!' and the investigator's being a likeable kind of person is not a reason for others to accept the hypothesis. It is in this sense that science is impersonal and objective. The reasons that can be offered for the acceptance or rejection of hypotheses are not dependent on particular persons. Experimental outcomes are reasons for acceptance or rejection; it does not matter who does the experiments, and if there is any query about them they can be done again in different places by different people. (see Popper, 1963, Introduction and Chapters 1 and 3; Magee, 1973).

Many of the things one will affirm in moral discussion are unprovable. However, we can now see that this is not something that divides moral thinking from scientific thinking. Equally, 'Trust me!' is not a good reason in moral discussion. If Mary has moral qualms and Anne wants her to set them aside but can think of nothing better to say than 'Trust me!', then Mary should stick to her qualms. Suppose Anne really does think that Mary is mistaken in objecting to Anne's proposal. Then in almost all cases there will be something that Anne could say that would set out why Anne thinks Mary is mistaken. (Often Anne will be badly placed to put it into words herself. An important aim of ethics courses – and of this book – is to enable people to develop a vocabulary with which to put moral hunches, reservations, qualms, etc. into words.) Once it has been set out it is no longer Anne-dependent. It is in the public domain. It can be appraised as a reason by anyone. It can be improved upon, amended and developed by others. How good or poor it is as a reason has nothing to do with its being Anne's. Thus, as far as impersonality is concerned, we need not suppose that moral discussion is different in kind from scientific discussion.

Sometimes the discussion of a moral issue can become very tangled, with quite different lines of argument getting knotted together. Then a cool analytical approach is invaluable. Such an approach is not less at home in moral than in scientific enquiry. Again, it is important in both areas to be able to articulate reasons and to be able to appraise reasons without being influenced by the fact that the reasons came from one person rather than another. And just as scientific thinking involves logic and experiment, moral thinking involves logic and thought experiment.

Morality and science are of course distinct. But we need not suppose that moral thinking is different from scientific thinking in the sense of involving steps of a kind that would be improper in the context of scientific reasoning.

1.6 OBJECTIVITY AND PARTICIPATION

We have suggested that there is no opposition between moral thinking and scientific thinking. However, a scientific orientation can lead us to view things in a way that makes some important matters harder to see clearly. Dwelling upon the breathtaking advances in scientific understanding of the world can lead to our seeing only what has been called the view from nowhere (cf. Nagel, 1986, pp. 3–9). A scientific account of climate or rock strata or nutrition or human development is supposed to be free from the distortions that would result if the matter were being looked at from the point of view of a particular person or group of persons or even a particular culture. To the extent that such an account turns out to be influenced by the preoccupations or interests of some person or group or culture, the account is regarded as imperfect and in need of improvement. For example, to the extent that psychoanalysis turns out to have been shaped by Freud's standpoint as a man, it has to be reconsidered and thought through again from a gender-neutral standpoint. What scientific enquiry aspires to is an understanding of its subject matter that is equally valid no matter what standpoint that subject matter is viewed from. To the extent that we see things scientifically, then, we see them as though we did not occupy one point of view rather than another. We see them as though we were looking at them from nowhere.

1.6a THE OBJECTIVE ATTITUDE

We also view them in an especially detached way. When we are trying to find out about climate or rock strata or nutrition we adopt or maintain an uninvolved, disengaged attitude to things. This detachment is characterstic of what has sometimes been called the **objective** attitude. It is the attitude of a spectator who watches what is going on but remains separate from it. The objective attitude does not rule out physical intervention. As well as looking at something, one might also poke at it (to take samples, or to see what happens next). However, one cannot greet it or exchange glances with it while still maintaining the objective attitude.

We may adopt the objective attitude towards another person. We then regard the other person as just another item in the physical world. People are regarded in this way when they are seen as objects of social policy, as subjects for treatment, as things to be taken into account and perhaps to be wary of, 'to be managed or handled or cured or trained' (Strawson, 1982). The objective attitude is one we might adopt if a person has a fit, or if we have some unavoidable dealings with someone we know to be awkward and quarrelsome, or if we realize that the person we are dealing with is simply being unreasonable once in a while. Then we relate to them, for the moment, as we might relate to something that was not a person at all: we try to make use of whatever information we have about what effects a given action of ours is likely to have, and we choose our actions accordingly. Equally we may sometimes sense that another person is taking the objective attitude towards us and is regarding us with detachment as a curiosity or as a specimen or as a case.

1.6b THE PARTICIPANT ATTITUDE

We are all familiar with a different way of relating to someone, which may be called the **participant** attitude. If a quarrel or argument is going on between two people and I am one of them then I am as much a participant as the other person is. Instead of being a detached spectator, I am involved and my involvement is of the same kind as the other person's. Also I remain in my personal viewpoint and do not seek to see things as though from some impersonal viewpoint, distinct from my personal one. Further, in recognizing the other person as like me, I view that person as also having a personal viewpoint. Seeing the other people I interact with as having their own viewpoints, I grasp that in their experience they are at the centre of the world just as I am at the centre of the world in my experience. In the participant attitude I take different personal viewpoints seriously, whereas in the objective attitude I seek to view everything as though from one impersonal viewpoint. Thus, whereas the objective attitude is characterized by detachment and an impersonal viewpoint, the participant attitude is characterized by involvement, a personal viewpoint, and a recognition of others' personal viewpoints.

When in the participant attitude, then, we see things from our own personal point of view (and do not attempt to view them as though from a neutral point of view which is not that of any person); we also see the other persons with whom we interact as having personal viewpoints of their own (rather than just as items fitting into the view seen from our viewpoint).

The difference between the participant attitude and the objective attitude is not fundamentally that one attitude is emotional and the other is unemotional. However, there are feelings that are characteristic of the participant attitude and are not compatible with the objective attitude. These include resentment, gratitude, forgiveness and anger (cf. Strawson, 1982, p. 62). It is only to the extent that I have the participant attitude towards another being – and thus am involved, remain in a personal viewpoint and view the other as having a personal viewpoint too – that I can have feelings like that. To the extent that my attitude towards someone is the participant attitude, if they hurt me I will normally be angry and indignant, and if they are kind to me I will feel grateful. (The presence of such feelings may show me that I was not as objective as I liked to think.) The objective attitude excludes such feelings; it may be an entirely dispassionate attitude, but it need not be:

> The objective attitude may be emotionally toned in many ways, but not in all ways: it may include repulsion or fear, it may include pity or even love, though not all kinds of love.
>
> (Strawson, 1982, p. 66)

Commenting on this passage, Daniel Dennett suggests that solicitude such as that 'of a gardener for his flowers' is also consistent with the objective attitude (Dennett, 1982, p. 158).

1.6c OBJECTIVE AND PARTICIPANT ATTITUDES

The objective attitude may sometimes be hard to sustain. If one senses that one is being mocked or taunted by a person, one may find oneself shifting from a stance of clinical detachment to one of involvement in a quarrel. In that case one no longer has the objective attitude but has the participant attitude instead.

The participant attitude, too, can be hard to sustain. If for a long while one has been in the participant attitude with regard to something and has detected no sign of the attitude's being reciprocated, one might find oneself having to shift from the participant attitude to the objective attitude. As we shall see in Chapter Three, this has implications for how the concept of care is to be understood.

Any but the most fleeting interpersonal relationship will typically involve a mixture of participant and objective attitudes. If the participant attitude goes unnoticed or unacknowledged, then the understanding of that relationship will be distorted; the distortion can then go on to affect the relationship itself. Strawson (1982) suggests that the objective attitude is available as a resource (for example, 'as a refuge . . . from the strains of involvement', p. 67). But there is a risk that, instead of being a resource which we may choose to make use of, it may lead to distortion of human interactions.

In a sense we each know how to relate to others while taking the participant attitude to them. This is knowledge that we all have. But those who come to talk and think in a professional way can be in danger of forgetting, overlooking, or losing sight of, that knowledge (cf. Strawson, 1982, p. 64) to the extent that officially approved, professional ways of talking are tailored to the objective attitude. There are people who are capable of love and friendship and yet who come to think that love or friendship is a set of techniques or a set of skills. They are then overlooking an important dimension of ordinary life. If when thinking about our life we systematically fail to see and draw upon important aspects of that life, our thinking is bound to be inadequate. So it is vital to leave room at the theoretical or conceptual or reflective level for the participant attitude to be taken into account. (These matters are discussed at length in Martin Buber's difficult but rewarding book *I and Thou*, 1958.)

We have noted that having the participant attitude towards someone is not a matter of feelings. Let us note also that it is not straightforwardly a matter of morality. In contrasting the participant and objective attitudes, we are not saying that morality calls upon us to treat some of the things in the world with special gentleness and solicitude and attention to their sensations and that treating them thus is having the participant attitude to them. Nor are we saying that taking the participant attitude to a person is *respecting* that person and is something that morality requires of us. (Taking the participant attitude with regard to someone is consistent with treating them in insulting or hurtful or harmful ways.) The point is rather that some important moral considerations can be satisfactorily grasped only in the context of a way of thinking that can accommodate the participant attitude. Calling attention to this attitude is not yet saying how people should treat each other; but some points about how people should treat each other are hard to make sense of unless one is alert to the participant attitude.

Treating a delicate, fragile object with great caution and gentleness so as to avoid breaking it is still treating it (rightly) as a thing. Treating patients as persons is not a matter of treating them with caution and gentleness in that way. There is a world of difference between the specific range of responses that are appropriate to persons and the responses that are appropriate only to things. In bringing attention to the perfectly familiar mode of interaction that people adopt in relating unreflectively to one another, we hope to make nurses alive to the possibility of drawing on that in the professional role. Of course most nurses already do draw on that. The point is that no one need have a sneaking sense that it is unscientific or unbusinesslike or unprofessional to do so; they need have no worry that increasingly professional work entails minimizing human contact.

1.7 FEELINGS IN MORAL DISCUSSION

Feelings plainly do have a place in the processes by which a person arrives at moral conclusions. Suppose I think that people ought not to speak disrespectfully of the recent dead. If a companion of mine makes mocking jokes about a recently dead person, thereby inviting my acquiescence in disrespectful talk, I am likely to have certain feelings – feelings of uneasiness and perhaps of anger. If, in order to avoid friction, I do not make plain my nonendorsement of such talk, then I shall feel compromised. Having feelings of certain kinds in situations of certain kinds is part and parcel of having moral views.

Sometimes a feeling of uneasiness about a course of action is one's first intimation that the action might be morally questionable. On feeling uneasy about it one may then pause to think about it and come to see reason for not doing it. (For example, you might be on the point of passing on recently acquired information about an acquaintance's love life. A momentary sense that you should not gossip makes you pause and wonder whether the acquaintance would prefer the story not to go too far. A moment's reflection leaves you with two or three reasons for keeping it to yourself.) Or one may voice the feeling to a companion, so that both wonder together for a moment whether there is indeed some reason for not acting in the way they envisaged. The outcome of this may be that some convincing reason comes to light; or it may be that no such reason appears and the feeling is dismissed.

So feelings can have the relatively humble role of prompting us to look for reasons. A grander role may be claimed for feelings. Suppose two people are arguing about an important issue. Perhaps the issue is whether the prolonging of life is always a top priority. Helen thinks that a patient should always be resuscitated if it is possible. Helen's reasons look pretty convincing. Andrew thinks that sometimes a person who could be resuscitated should not be. He has offered various reasons for this, but Helen has had a plausible answer for each of them. It looks as though, as far as this discussion session is concerned, Helen is right and Andrew is wrong. At this point Andrew may say 'Well, that's all well and good, but I just feel that resuscitation is sometimes wrong'. This is in effect a declaration that, despite the apparent weight of reasons. Andrew is not going to change his position.

Perhaps Andrew suspects that there are important considerations which have not come out in their discussion. This may be a very reasonable suspicion, and he may be wise to suspend judgement until there is an opportunity to explore such further considerations.

But it may also be that Andrew is invoking his feeling as a justification for not going along with the conclusion that all the arguments seem to favour. In this book we wish to stress that feelings do not have such a role in rational discussion. Feelings do not justify people in sticking to moral views which are not defensible by reasons. So, if Andrew claims to be justified by his feelings in rejecting the view that Helen has given him overwhelming reasons for accepting, Helen is entitled to deny such justification.

Of course, Andrew may choose to reject Helen's carefully and thoroughly argued view without claiming to be justified in rejecting it and without waiting to see whether some so far unthought-of reasons will later come to light. Then he is being unreasonable. But he is entitled to be unreasonable if he wants to.

In short, if Andrew claims to be justified by a feeling in refusing to accept a conclusion that is supported by decisive arguments, then Andrew is simply wrong; feelings don't justify in that way. If Andrew refuses to go along with the conclusion for the moment, suspecting that there may be more relevant arguments than the ones that have so far come to light, the matter is left open for further enquiry – perhaps at a later stage. If Andrew refuses to go along with the conclusion but neither claims the justification of feelings nor anticipates possible reasons – which just happen not yet to be available – then he is being unreasonable.

Sometimes it is thought that each of us simply has certain feelings about what is right or wrong in a given situation, and all a person needs to do is take note of his or her own moral feelings and, if appropriate, put them into words; beyond that there is nothing to be said. This is a mistake. It is far from being the case that in moral matters we have to be governed by inarticulate feelings. As we shall see, there is in most cases a very great deal that can relevantly be said about a moral problem. And being able to understand, analyse and discuss problems of professional morality is part of what is involved in being a professional.

We have suggested that feelings are not to be given the function of 'stop' signs in reasonable discussion. We should also note that feelings are not fixed and unchangeable. Feelings of fear, suspicion, or hostility towards people of another race or religion can disappear as a result of mixing with such people. Such feelings can also come into existence if one comes to be persuaded that such people constitute a threat to a cherished way of life. When in the course of calm, rational discussion one comes to have moral views which one did not previously have, one is likely also to acquire feelings about the matters to which those moral views relate.

TWO

Moral deliberation

2.1 ELEMENTS OF ETHICAL DELIBERATION

A practical decision is a decision as to what to do. The process of thinking that produces a practical decision is known as deliberation. At the start of a piece of deliberation, a person is undecided as to which of several courses of action to take. Where the selecting or non-selecting of one of those courses of action is seen as depending on moral considerations, the deliberation is moral deliberation (or ethical deliberation; we take the terms 'moral' and 'ethical' to be interchangeable). Deliberation might be interrupted, or the person may just give up thinking about the problem; but if neither of these things happens then the deliberation ends with the selection of a course of action. The selected course of action might not be one of the ones originally considered; she might have rejected all of those and thought of another course of action altogether.

Ethical deliberation can be viewed as involving the following elements:

- moral principles
- an appreciation of the situation
- a review of possible courses of action
- application of the principles
- decision (selection of one of the practical possibilities).

Just for illustrative purposes, let us look at a simplified fragment of deliberation. We take once again the example given at the beginning of Chapter One. A patient says to you 'Am I going to die, nurse?' You have no reason to think he will live through the night. You could say 'Oh, there's plenty of life in you yet.' Or you could try to think of another response. You have always believed that lying is wrong. Your thinking might go something like this:

1. It is wrong to lie.
2. To say to this patient now 'There's plenty of life in you' is to lie.
3. So to say to this patient now 'there's plenty of life in you' is wrong.
4. So I won't do that.
5. So I'll try to think of something else.

This is a simplified fragment. It is a fragment in that a piece of thinking like this would always be embedded in a larger process of thinking which would involve the selection of the lying principle from among other principles and would also involve the selection of other principles and their being brought to bear on the situation in a similar way. And it is simplified in that applying a principle's key concept to a possible course of action in the situation (the concept of lying, at line 2) and then applying the principle to that course of action to arrive at a judgement about it (at line 3) and then arriving at a decision (at line 4) are presented as though they were simple straightforward steps.

However, simplified and fragmentary though the example is, it does contain the elements noted above. There is a moral principle (noted at line 1). There is an appreciation of the situation: you size up the situation as including a patient claiming a response from you and as including the unlikelihood of that patient's surviving the night. (No doubt this appreciation could be developed or filled out. In general there will be scope for a fuller appreciation of a situation and for reconsidering the appreciation so far arrived at. Often, though, the pressing need for a swift decision will rule out a protracted process of situation-appreciation.) There is a review of possible courses of action: say 'there's plenty of life in you yet' or think of something else. (Plainly this is not an exhaustive review: in any case of deliberation some sort of review is present even if it is a very cursory or hasty one.) There is an application of principle to a possible course of action: the suitability of a certain course of action for the no-lying principle to apply to it is highlighted (line 2) and a moral judgement is arrived at (line 3). There is a decision (line 4).

2.2. STAGES OF DELIBERATION

When deliberation occurs, there are background factors which the person deliberating brings with her to the situation. These include general principles and values and beliefs about the world. They do not have to be thought of as unshakeable, but they do not usually come into question in the context of ordinary practical deliberation. More will be said about these factors below. In the present section we distinguish a number of different stages of deliberation. For the sake of clarity we shall leave certain complications out of account to start with. They can be introduced later.

The stages of deliberation and the order in which they occur are as follows:

1. Appreciation of the situation and possible outcomes.
2. Review of possible courses of action.
3. Selection and application of principles.
4. Weighing of practical considerations.
5. Decision.

Stage 1 is a matter of taking in the facts of the situation and seeing some as more central and important and others as more marginal and unimportant. (Suppose you have described a situation *fully*. The aspects you consider more marginal and unimportant are the ones you would leave out if you were asked to give a shorter description of the situation.) Stage 1 also involves grasping how the situation is going to develop. (Perhaps the situation is a stable one and things are just going to stay the same; perhaps there are processes going on that will lead to changes unless someone intervenes.)

Stage 2 is a matter of noticing the various courses of action that could be taken.

Stage 3 is important. A person may have quite a lot of principles, and some may be relevant to the situation while others may not. In deliberation, a person may select some of her principles and bring them to bear on the situation and leave others out of consideration. For a principle to be brought to bear on the situation, a link needs to be found between the principle and some aspect of the situation or of one of the possible courses of action. Thus, in the schematic example of section 2.1, the link was made by means of the concept of lying. The concept features in the no-lying principle. Because of the facts of the situation (here the fact that the patient is going to die soon, a fact noted at stage 1) that concept also applies to one of the possible courses of action: saying 'there's plenty of life in you' is a possible course of action, and it is an instance of lying. Thus the no-lying principle, once selected, can be connected up to that possible course of action.

At stage 4, note is taken of reasons for taking or for not taking each of the various possible courses of action. Some actions are of a kind that is usually wrong, and that is a reason not to take them. Some actions have bad consequences and that is a reason not to take them. Some actions have good consequences, and that is a reason to take them. Sometimes a reason for a person not to take a certain course of action is that they do not want to be the kind of person who does things like that. In our schematic example one reason for not saying 'there's plenty of life in you', was *that saying it would be wrong*. This reason resulted from the application of the no-lying principle. We classify reasons of this kind – reasons about things being right or wrong or obligatory, etc. – as considerations of duty, and they are discussed below. Other kinds of reasons coming into stage 4, and discussed below, are considerations of value and of character (virtue and vice). Considerations of duty, and perhaps others too, may be based on general principles as in the example considered. But one may also find that some reasons for or against an action are hard to relate to general principles.

Stage 5 is a matter of deciding on a stage 2 course of action in the light of the considerations noted at stage 4. Sometimes one consideration is a decisive reason to rule out a certain course of action straight away. Or it may be that one consideration leaves one with no choice but to take a certain course of action regardless of what the other possible courses of action are. More often, though, there will be one or more courses of action which there are some reasons for taking and some reasons for not taking. Then the deliberating person has to take due account of all those reasons and try to see which are most important. It may be that there is some reason for acting in a certain way, but also an important reason not to let that first reason be decisive. Thus there may be good reason not to give much weight to reasons of one's own personal convenience.

Just as there is no foolproof way of gaining knowledge (see section 1.5 above) so there is no foolproof way of deliberating and deciding. There is scope for error at each of the stages of deliberation. At stage 1 some feature of the situation may be simply overlooked, a marginal fact may be taken for a central one, and so on. At stage 2, possibilities of action can be overlooked; some possibilities of action are likely to be noticed only by a person of great ingenuity and resourcefulness; again, someone might think they see a possibility of action where there really is not one. At stage 3 one may fail to see a way in which a link could be made between the situation or the options and some moral principle. (Thus one might sincerely embrace the principle of loving one's neighbour but fail to see some unfortunate person as one's neighbour; in this way a principle might not be applied even though it could have been.) At stage 4 some considerations might go unnoticed, one might mistakenly suppose there to be a certain duty or one might incorrectly judge the value of some outcome (see section 2.3b, below). Finally, in deciding on a course of action one can go wrong in such ways as being unduly moved by a relatively unimportant consideration or being unable to keep all the relevant considerations in view at the same time.

To be practical and realistic, we have to take account of human error. Since there is room for error or distortion at each stage of deliberation,

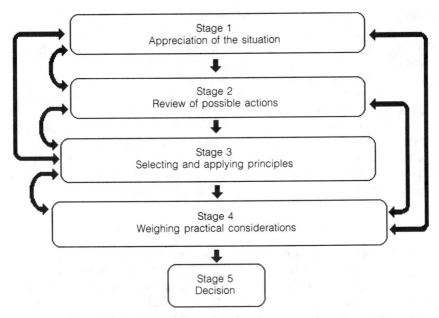

Figure 2.2 The five stages of moral deliberation and their interrelationships.

we should not be too confident at a later stage that everything has been got right at earlier stages. Each earlier stage can be revisited from later stages, illustrated in Figure 2.2. In seeking to apply a principle at stage 3 we may come to notice things previously overlooked at stage 1 and thus modify the stage 1 appreciation. Again, at stage 4 it may turn out that each of the practical options already noted is unacceptable; this may lead to a return to stage 2 to see whether a greater exercise of imagination and ingenuity will reveal practical options which were not noticed the first time round.

Apart from being ready to revisit earlier stages, we may do well to use the help of others when it is available; another person will often recognize one's mistakes or oversights more readily than one will oneself. And one may be well advised to be alert to facts about oneself (weaknesses, preoccupations, prejudices, etc.) that could lead to distortion (cf. Shelly, 1980, p. 36).

2.3 MORAL AND EVALUATIVE CONSIDERATIONS

Many considerations can feature in stage 4 of moral deliberation and discussion – considerations about treachery, loyalty, friendship, considerations about relationships ('you can't just gossip about a colleague to outsiders'; 'maybe you should send a Get Well card just because she's a classmate, even if she isn't a special friend'), considerations about theft, self-respect, candour, gratitude, and so on. The aim of this section is to highlight four distinct groups of considerations which feature in different ways in stage 4 and related discussion. Clarity about these considerations and how they are related to each other can help with the appraisal of some of the moral arguments that will be considered later. The considerations to be reviewed are those of duty, value, virtue and rights. Considerations of duty bear directly on the question 'What am I to do?', considerations of value on the question 'What am I to cherish?' considerations of virtue on the question 'What am I to be?' and considerations of rights on the question 'What am I to respect?' Considerations of all these groups can bear upon the selection of a course of action at stage 5.

2.3a STAGE 4 CONSIDERATIONS – DUTY

We often speak of someone having a duty to do something, and we mean that morality requires the person to do that thing. The point that we are then making can be put in other words. We can say that the person ought to do that thing, or that the person has an obligation to do that thing, or that it would be wrong for the person not to do that thing. We use the notion of obligation and the related notions of right and wrong conduct, of duty, and of what a person ought to do when our focus is on actions that someone has done or might do. These notions are sometimes called **deontic** notions. Part of a person's concern, when she reflects morally, is to answer questions like 'What am I to do?' and 'What should the charge nurse have done?' And deontic notions are likely to feature in her reflection. When a moral statement is best expressed in terms of obligation, it is a statement about conduct, about how some person should or should not behave.

2.3b STAGE 4 CONSIDERATIONS – VALUE

Whereas considerations of duty have to do with conduct, value has to do with objects or states of affairs and with the question 'What am I to cherish?' If a certain action will bring about a valuable state of affairs, that is a reason for taking that course of action. If a course of action will bring about a state of affairs with negative value – a bad state of affairs – that is a reason for not taking that course of action.

We make a value judgement every time we treat something as worth having and every time we think that some state of affairs is worth bringing about. Likewise, taking things to be not worth bringing about is making value judgements. And we make comparative value judgements when we treat something as less worth having than something else or as worth giving up for the sake of something else. If you buy a pair of gloves for £ 4.00, you are judging that having the gloves is of more value to you than the things that you would have been able to do with the £ 4.00 otherwise. If you spend an evening working for examinations instead of going out to the pictures, you are judging that the improvement of your chances in the examination is more important than the enjoyment of that evening out. Sometimes people make mistakes about value – perhaps through carelessness or thoughtlessness. Many folk tales warn us against such carelessness. The story of King Midas is a case in point. On being given the chance to have whatever he wished, King Midas wished that everything he touched would turn to gold. He judged, unthinkingly, that gold is always more worth having than anything else. When his breakfast and his children turned to gold, however, he found out that he had been mistaken and that there are more valuable breakfasts and children than golden ones.

Is value a purely personal matter? The Midas story suggests that it is not. It is not just that Midas happened (without realizing it) to value organic breakfasts and children more then metallic ones; anyone could be expected to make the same judgement. And if someone did not, would that person not just be mistaken? This is the mark of impersonal value. If one thing is impersonally more valuable than another, then anyone who thinks otherwise is mistaken. Of course, any of us may be mistaken in his or her judgements of impersonal value but we can tell whether one of our judgements is a judgement of impersonal value by considering how we would respond to someone who did not share our value judgement. Suppose a man gives a big place to early jazz in his way of life. He spends a significant proportion of his earnings on records and literature about them, on visits to New Orleans and similar items. He spends much of his leisure time listening to the music, reading about it, entering into controversies with other enthusiasts, and the like. He has neither the money nor the time to go to classical concerts, buy records of classical music, etc. as well as pursuing his interest in early jazz. In pursuing that interest to the exclusion of classical music, he is treating early jazz as having greater importance than classical music. Now, if he also thinks that people who do not give a similar priority to early jazz are mistaken, then the comparative value judgement he is making is a judgement of impersonal value. (No doubt it is an incorrect judgement, but that is another matter.) But if he does not think that those who go to classical concerts are mistaken then his assignment of such an important place in his life to early jazz is a matter of personal value.

So a thing is of value to the extent that it is worth having, worth pursuing, worth going to trouble and expense for. It is of impersonal value if anyone who fails to treat it as worth having, etc. is mistaken. It is of personal value to a person if it has an important place in that person's conception of how they want their life to be. A thing can be of (personal) value to someone without being of the same impersonal value.

We do well to try to improve our views about what is of value and what is of greater or less value. This holds both for personal values and for impersonal ones. There is no reason to suppose that people are generally clear about what really matters most to them. And there is certainly no reason to suppose that people's views about what is of impersonal value are beyond improvement.

An element of nursing ethics is respecting the values of others. Part of what is at issue here is fallibility about impersonal values. Each of us can be wrong about all sorts of things, and one of the sorts of things we can be wrong about is impersonal values. Thinking that something is impersonally valuable is thinking that anyone who disagrees is mistaken. But in such a case I may be the one who is mistaken. We need to beware of giving insufficient credence to that possibility. The possibility of being mistaken is present also in the case of personal values. (People sometimes think that wealth is what matters most to them and then discover that they were wrong.) But in addition there is there the possibility of imposing one's own values on someone else. When that happens, a choice that may well be the best one in the light of one person's personal values is implemented for another person.

Questions of value are not in themselves moral questions. A state of affairs in which many people are suddenly dead or injured is a bad state of affairs whether it is due to human agency or to natural causes. Its being due to natural causes or human agency makes no difference to its negative value but may make a very great difference to other questions such as questions of duty and of character.

2.3c STAGE 4 CONSIDERATIONS – VIRTUE

Virtue has to do with character and with the question 'What am I to be?' A consideration entering into stage 4 of deliberation might be that to act in a certain way would be cruel or arrogant. Then the person's reason for not acting in that way is that they do not want to be a cruel person or an arrogant person. That is not the kind of person they want to be.

For some reason, the word 'virtue' seems to have fallen into disuse. It is used fairly infrequently and when it is used it can sound priggish or pompous. And yet we think and talk in terms of virtues and vices a very great deal. All the time, as we get to know someone, we are getting impressions of the kind of person they are; and often we are deciding in the light of that whether we want to get to know them better or not. Suppose I discover that a friend of mine knows the person I am going to be working for from next week; the first thing I ask will be 'What's she like?' I might be told that she is kind, understanding, loyal, firm, sympathetic; I might be told that she is vindictive, a ditherer, moody, devious, shifty, a bully. Some of these qualities are virtues, some are defects or vices. The fact that we usually have little difficulty telling which are which shows that thinking in terms of virtues and vices is nothing strange or unusual.

The way to make progress towards becoming the kind of person one wants to be is to act as the kind of person one wants to be would act. So the fact that a person of the kind we want to be would take a certain course of action in the present situation is a reason for us to take that course of action. And the fact that a person of a kind we want not to be would take a certain course of action is a reason for us not to take that course of action. That is how considerations of virtue and vice enter into stage 4 of deliberation. Virtue and vice also relate to the concerns of this book in other ways, as we shall see in section 2.6, below.

2.3d STAGE 4 CONSIDERATIONS – RIGHTS

This once unfashionable concept is forcing itself upon our attention ever more in recent years. Rights often act as a counterbalance to value. It may often appear that a person's preferences or interests should be set aside in view of something of great value or importance that can be achieved at their expense. When we talk of individuals having rights we mean that their interests or preferences may not be overridden even to achieve great value. For example, when we say a patient has a right to decline to take part in drug trials, we mean that the patient's merely not wanting to take part is enough to make it wrong to proceed with trials involving that patient. The patient's refusal does not have to be justifiable; the risk or discomfort does not have to be great or even noticeable. When we say that a wealthy lawyer has the right of ownership of a certain expensive coat, we mean that her wanting to hold on to it is good enough reason for her being allowed to do so even if some poorer person is in greater need of a coat and a better (more valuable) state of affairs would exist if the poor person had the coat instead. If we say an unborn baby has a right to life, we are denying that the question whether it should live or not depends only on how happy or unhappy its birth is going to make people. If we say that a person has a right not to be physically encumbered for several months through the failure of a properly used and usually reliable product, we are claiming that in such a case a woman's preference to be no longer pregnant is a reason for condoning an abortion. If we say that a person has a right to health care we are saying that there is reason for that person to receive health care even if greater value could be brought about by directing resources elsewhere.

In general, the notion of a right functions in moral deliberation in such a way as to make moral issues turn not just on how much or how little value various ways of acting will produce. Much action is intended to lead to greater value. Metaphorically, we can think of the contemplated value as being ahead and of the person who acts as moving towards it. In terms of this metaphor, rights can be thought of as side constraints; they do not set us goals which we are to achieve; their role in moral deliberation is rather to set limits on the paths that we may choose to move along towards whatever goals we pursue (cf. Nozick, 1988).

We need not here decide the question whether rights are absolute or can be overridden by other considerations provided the other considerations are sufficiently powerful. Thus it might be argued that if the goal to be achieved is of enormous and uncontested value and is extremely likely to be achieved provided some right is set aside then transgressing the side constraints set by rights is justifiable. The important thing for present purposes is not to settle this question but to be clear about the distinctive character of rights (especially the difference between them and values) and to be able to recognize considerations about rights when they come into the discussion of a problem.

2.4 PRINCIPLES

Principles are conduct-guiding generalizations, designating certain kinds of considerations as reasons for acting in certain ways or for not acting in certain ways. At stage 3 of deliberation, a person selects one or more principles as relevant to the situation and brings those principles to bear on the situation or the practical options. On being thus applied, each principle will then give a reason for action. (Because of the no-lying principle, the fact that saying 'there is plenty of life in you' is a lie becomes a reason for not saying it.) A principle will carry weight with a person and shape that person's decisions only if the person believes in the principle or subscribes to it. It is common in discussions of health care ethics to make frequent reference to a small number of principles and to take it that those principles are appropriate ones for people working in health care to subscribe to and that they are especially basic and widely applicable. (Such principles are considered at length in Beauchamp and Childress, 1983.)

One of these is the principle of beneficence. The word 'beneficence' may seem a strange one. It is akin to 'benevolence'. A benevolent action is one which is intended to bring about good consequences (it is well-willing). A beneficent action is one which actually does bring about good consequences (it is well-doing). The principle of beneficence urges us to do beneficent actions. According to this principle, the fact that a certain action would bring about human good, either in general or to particular persons (such as the patient currently in one's care) is a moral reason for deciding on that action.

There is also a principle of nonmaleficence. A maleficent action is one which brings about bad consequences. The principle of nonmaleficence urges us not to do maleficent actions; according to it, the fact that a certain action would bring about human harm, either in general or to particular persons (such as present patients) is a moral reason for deciding against that action.

There is obviously some kinship between those two principles. Indeed, many would say that they are not really distinct principles at all and that nonmaleficence is already covered by beneficence. However, it might be argued that the obligation not to harm people is more stringent than the obligation to do good to people and that, hence, the obligation not to harm people must be founded on a more urgent principle (cf. Harman, 1977, pp. 110–111).

The principles of beneficence and nonmaleficence lead to duties to act in ways that will produce value (or prevent negative value). The principles thus connect the idea of duty with that of value. There is another principle which is known both as the principle of respect for persons and as the principle of autonomy. It owes its central position in modern ethical thought to Immanuel Kant (1785). It may be expressed thus: do not use a person merely as a means. It says in effect that, if a certain course of action would involve using a person merely as a means, that is a powerful reason for not taking that course of action.

Let us pause here to review the notions of means and end. Very often when a person acts, they do so because they have some end which they want to achieve. An end is the same as a goal or a purpose or an aim. It is rarely the case that one's end can be achieved in one step. Often what one does is not bring about one's end directly but rather bring about something else which will then cause one's end to come about (or help to cause it). This something else is then a means to an end. For example, I may want to be drinking a cup of coffee. Then my drinking a cup of coffee is an end of mine. I boil a kettle. I have no special pleasure in boiling kettles. But the boiling of the kettle will help to bring it about that I am drinking a cup of coffee. Boiling the kettle is then a means to having a cup of coffee. Objects and implements can also be called means. Thus the kettle itself is a means to my end, on this occasion and on many others.

The same thing can be sometimes a means and sometimes an end. In the above example, my drinking a cup of coffee was an end. I just wanted to enjoy that flavour, that texture, that temperature. On another occasion

I may drink a cup of coffee in the hope that it will help me to stay awake. Then drinking the coffee is a means to the end of staying awake.

Let us return to the Kantian principle: do not use a person merely as a means. A moment's reflection should satisfy the reader that most people are using other people as means a lot of the time. Every time you get a shop assistant to help you you are using the shop assistant as a means to your end. Further reflection should satisfy the reader that if people stopped using one another as means altogether, life would be massively less convenient and comfortable than it is.

But notice the word 'merely'. The principle of respect or autonomy does not rule out using people as means; it only rules out using them merely as means. As a thinking, acting being I am a source of plans; I make plans, form aspirations, entertain ambitions, think out projects. Some I simply abandon; some I shelve for reconsideration later (perhaps for reconsideration only when I realize that the time left to me is short); some I try to combine with one another, perhaps making adjustments, until I have a plan I want to implement. My plans for a year or a week or a day may be thought out in great detail or may be only very roughly sketched. In the example above, having a cup of coffee came into my plan. That part of the plan I executed, and I made use of the kettle as a means in the course of doing so. The kettle is not a thinking, acting being. It has no plans, aspirations, ambitions, projects, unfinished business. My conscripting the kettle into my plans did not interfere with the implementation of any plan that the kettle had, and I was not demeaning the kettle by treating its plans as of no account. I was treating the kettle as a means, but not violating any moral requirement in so doing.

What the respect/autonomy principle rules out is using a person merely as a means in the way that I used the kettle merely as a means. The kettle really was there just for my convenience. So it was all right to use it as though it was there just for my convenience. It does not have any convenience of its own. But no person is there just for my convenience. They each have their own convenience. Even if they are there for my convenience (at the hairdresser's, say), they are not there only for my convenience. To return to the shop assistant, he has plans, ambitions, aspirations, projects, unfinished business of various kinds. He is as much a source of plans as I am. There is nothing that makes me, as a source of plans, more important than he is. The world of nature is not waiting to have my plans implemented in it rather than his. I am no more entitled to take it for granted that his plans are of no account and that he is there only to feature in my plans than he is entitled to take it for granted that my plans are of no account and that I am there only to feature in his plans.

In fact, it is unlikely that much of the shop assistant's plans will come to light during our brief interaction. But in the shop assistant case, unlike the kettle case, the autonomy/respect principle requires me not to conscript the assistant into my plans in a way which treats his own plans as of no account. An extreme way of doing that would be to shoot the shop assistant dead in the course of carrying out a plan to rob the shop. Another extreme violation of the principle is slavery. The slave is used in the implementation of the slave-owner's plans in a way that treats the slave as having no plans that are of any account. This is so even if the slave-owner is a disinterested philanthropist who has conscripted the slave into a plan which will not benefit the slave-owner at all but will benefit the rest of mankind immensely. Even if my plan is a plan to benefit you, the autonomy principle still forbids me to conscript you into my plan in a way that treats your own plans as of no account.

To treat what may be of importance to another person as of no account is to have contempt for that person. The principle under discussion requires us to have respect rather than contempt for all persons. That is why it is often called the principle of respect for persons. The aspect of persons that it latches on to, though, is in particular their capacity to live not by a blueprint programmed into them or by a set of rules thought up by someone else but by goals that they have set for themselves and by a life-plan and in a life-style that they have chosen for themselves. It latches on to the idea of persons as self-governing, and that is the point of its being called the principle of autonomy.

Beneficence and nonmaleficence are central to the enterprise of health care in a very obvious way. To remove or alleviate the suffering of disease and injury, to restore people to bodily health and well-being, to bring ease and comfort to those who cannot be cured are plainly aspects of beneficence. In recent years, the restoration of the patient to full autonomy has become more prominent than it previously was as an aim of health care, and there has been growing awareness of the need to consider implications of the patient's being an autonomous person. How the principles of autonomy and beneficence are to be balanced is a central issue, and it will be considered in Chapter 4.

In addition to beneficence and autonomy, people deliberating a moral issue may invoke justice. Identifying and formulating a definitive principle is harder here than in the other cases. Justice is the subject of a vast and often very difficult body of literature. Moreover, problems of justice in health care are not among the main issues dealt with in this book. Nevertheless, a brief discussion of justice is in order.

One principle which expresses an important part of the idea of justice is the principle that any two cases are to be treated alike unless they differ in some relevant respect. If one child has been allowed to stay up late, another child ought in the name of justice to be allowed to stay up late unless there is a relevant difference. (Presumably the second child's being two years younger than the first child is a relevant difference.) If a certain level of improvement is a reason for a patient's being discharged from hospital in one part of the country then that level of improvement is a reason for a patient's being discharged from hospital in another part of the country. If two people do comparable work or their work is of equal value then, in the name of justice, they ought to get comparable pay.

More specialized principles of justice may be identified to pick out types of relevant difference that frequently occur. Thus intensity of need, place in a queue, and importance to the community may all be factors relevant to treating some people more favourably than others. The important thing for us to note here is that, in any discussion of a proposal to treat apparently similar cases differently, the above principle of equal treatment places on those who advocate different treatment the burden of specifying some relevant difference between the cases. It will then be up to others to consider whether the specified difference really is relevant and of sufficient weight to satisfy the principle.

We have singled out these principles of beneficence, nonmaleficence, autonomy and justice for special attention because of their centrality and breadth of application. Much moral reasoning invokes considerations which are more specific and concrete than these, however, and we shall have occasion to mention many other principles in the following chapters.

2.5 TRADITIONS OF MORAL THOUGHT

We have stressed the importance of principles of beneficence and autonomy. Each of these is central to an important tradition of ethical thought. While the present book does not seek to be especially associated with either tradition, it is appropriate to acknowledge a debt to each of them.

Utilitarianism

Utilitarianism is a two-part doctrine: one part is that the rightness or wrongness of an act depends only on the value of its consequences; the other part is that that value is entirely a matter of happiness, pleasure or (in more sophisticated versions) preference-satisfaction. Unhappiness, pain or preference-frustration is negative value and has to be taken into account in reckoning the value of a state of affairs. Utilitarianism takes morality to be primarily about value and only derivatively about virtue, rights or duty (apart from the duty to maximize value).

According to utilitarianism there is ultimately only one duty, namely the duty to produce value. So stage 4 in utilitarian deliberation will not feature a lot of competing duties; the focus will rather be on considerations of value. The value that a course of action would produce is a reason for taking that course of action; the disvalue or negative value that it would produce is a reason for not taking it. A central question to be answered at stage 5 of utilitarian deliberation will be what value losses can be traded off against what value gains.

Consider again the example of sections 1.1 and 2.1. In a utilitarian perspective, lying would be considered wrong only to the extent that it led to bad consequences. The generalization that lying is wrong would be considered to have only limited validity. The most prominent considerations at stage 4 would be the value of the consequences of various courses of action that could be taken. The decisive consideration at stage 5 would be which action has the most valuable consequences; if the best consequences are to be achieved by lying, then stage 5 of utilitarian deliberation will produce a decision to lie.

Thus utilitarianism treats beneficence (understood in a particular way) – or beneficence-plus-nonmaleficence – as the whole story about morality. Morality is in the end a matter of acting rightly, and right action is a matter of acting in such a way as to maximize the value of the consequences. (Variants of utilitarianism involve various detailed accounts of what value consists in, but it is always a matter of pleasure, happiness or preference – satisfaction.) Sometimes it is convenient to speak of a moral argument that is based on the principle of beneficence as a utilitarian argument. When we speak in that way in this book we do not wish to suggest that no one but a utilitarian need take any notice of the argument; we mean merely to stress the fact that that argument, unlike some other ones, is available to people who take a utilitarian standpoint. Utilitarians and nonutilitarians alike subscribe to the principle of beneficence; the difference is that the utilitarians think it is the whole story.

Sometimes utilitarianism is charged with being at most part of the story about morality, not the whole story. One reason for suspecting that utilitarianism is not the whole story is that utilitarianism takes account only of what can be seen from an objective viewpoint whereas much of morality is importantly personal and needs the participant attitude. The kind of concern for one's fellow creatures that utilitarianism countenances is comparable to the solicitude of a gardener for his flowers or of a miser for her coins; it has a place in morality, but it is not adequate to take the place of the personal regard and concern that moral beings have for each other (cf. Dennett, 1982, p. 158, and section 1.7 above).

Kantian ethics

As formulated above, the principle of respect or autonomy is one version of Kant's Categorical Imperative. (Though perhaps less prominent in

Kant's own writings than other versions stressing the universalizability of moral imperatives, the respect/autonomy version is the version we shall emphasize in this book.) In articulating and exploring that principle, Kant made a lasting contribution to practical ethics. However, Kant's own theory of ethics was to the effect that the Categorical Imperative is the whole story about ethics. From a Kantian standpoint, a principle of beneficence is admissible as part of ethics only if it can be shown to conform with the Categorical Imperative. And any conflict between beneficence and autonomy would have to be resolved in favour of autonomy. Thus, to return once again to our example, a Kantian case could be made for saying that deceiving the patient, even for his own good (e.g. for his own piece of mind), would be using the patient merely as a means to a good state of affairs and would thus be wrong.

Readers of this book may not wish to embrace the Kantian view that respecting persons and not treating them merely as means constitutes the whole of morality. But it may still be found that considerations of the kind that Kant drew to our attention and which utilitarian thinking tends to obscure bear importantly on issues in health care ethics.

There are some moral deliberators who, without being committed to one of these traditions to the exclusion of the other, tend to give greater weight at stage 5 to the stage 4 reasons that are supported by the principles of beneficence and nonmaleficence; and there are others who tend to give greater weight to reasons supported by the principle of respect for persons. In Chapter Four we shall consider two models of moral decision-making which differ in the relative importance they attribute to beneficence-backed considerations.

2.6 DELIBERATION AND VIRTUE

In first presenting the stages of deliberation, we made some simplifying assumptions. One was that deliberation proceeds through the different stages in turn. We removed that simplifying assumption when we acknowledged that 'earlier' stages may be revisited after 'later' ones. Another simplifying assumption was that a person deliberating really does go through all the stages and think the corresponding thoughts. But often this does not happen at all, at least at a conscious level. A virtuous person will deliberate well without going painstakingly through the stages we have examined.

Virtue need involve no preoccupation with rules or explicitly formulated principles, (cf. Wiggins, 1978; McDowell, 1979). A virtuous person does not need to call to mind a moral rule saying 'be welcoming to newcomers'. For her, such rules are redundant; the situation where she is confronted with newcomers presents itself as one which calls for welcoming words and movements and she acts accordingly. It might be an effort – after a hard and grinding day; but it is not the kind of effort that would be involved in acting out of character. What in a sense is natural for a virtuous person may be against the grain for someone who is not virtuous or not yet virtuous. A not-yet-virtuous person may do well to bear in mind certain rules, especially if she is conscious of special weaknesses she has. If I have a tendency to humiliate the vulnerable, bearing in mind a rule might be the best way to combat that tendency. Moral development is in part a matter of responses coming to be second nature when previously they needed to be rule-backed.

Virtue is in part a matter of habits of conduct, in part a cognitive matter (a kind person is quick to detect another's unhappiness or unease, more generally a virtuous person will go wrong less than most of us in appreciating situations), in part a matter of having certain kinds of feeling and not other kinds, in part a matter of having certain concerns (such as a concern that others not suffer or be made foolish). An important aspect of virtue is that a virtuous person's first response is likely to be the same as her considered response. A person of impeccably sound moral views and in no way wicked may in moments of crisis or pressure or surprise say or do things which she later wishes she had not said or done. The unthinking response was not the response she would have wished to have. For a virtuous person, the unthinking response is one that, in the main, she does not regret or wish she could dissociate herself from.

Thus a person who is practised at deliberation and good at it will not laboriously rehearse all the stages we have considered every time they decide what to do. However, if asked to give an account of their decision, even they will have to set out something like the stages we have examined. If they are teaching others to do their moral thinking well, they will have to work through those stages. And if they have to advocate or defend a distinctive style of deliberation for their profession then they will once again have to articulate what is involved in deliberation.

There is an ancient debate as to whether virtue can be learnt or not. Without entering into that debate here we make the working assumption that to a great extent the virtues of nursing can be acquired. People are not born nurses. We shall see that becoming good at caring in the sense that is appropriate for nursing involves a number of virtues, although not the same ones as have traditionally been invoked (cf. Salvage, 1985, p. 5). And we shall see how deliberating well in nursing reflects those virtues.

THREE

Caring and being cared for

3.1 WHAT IS CARING?

'Care' is a simple word. But the concept it stands for turns out to be more complex. A care may be a worry, a burdened state of mind arising from fear, a doubt or a concern. To be charged with the care of someone or something is to be responsible for the well-being of that person or object. To care for someone is to supply protection and preservation. Care can be a feeling, concern or interest in something, providing food, being available, looking after someone or something.

Care involves another party. This may be an inanimate object, like a car or a piece of furniture, or it may be an animal. However, we most often think of caring as looking after the interests of another human being. This chapter is about the establishing of this relationship, and particularly the potential ethical issues it involves.

The above ideas are familiar and uncontroversial. This helps us to realize that the actions, thoughts and feelings associated with caring are familiar to each of us from our own experience. Indeed, many writers, both in philosophy and in nursing, regard caring as necessary for human existence. Without care and the ability to care, life as we know it would not be possible. A sense of security and of belonging, for example, could not exist. It does not follow, though, that caring is something we all instinctively know how to do.

To see this, consider Mr Smith and Mr Jones. They are both in their late 60s, proud family men, brought together because their wives happened to be admitted to the same hospital ward. Mrs Jones had been taken ill several months earlier. She had collapsed at home, was not able to move her legs, and could not speak. She still could not do much for herself now and this distressed Mr Jones each time he came to see her. In fact, he was finding it increasingly difficult to visit her; she was not the person he knew and loved and it took so much out of him to see her sometimes with particles of food drying at the side of her mouth, her eyes vacant, her mood tearful. His visits became more infrequent and when he did come to see his wife he kept his coat on as if he was just about to go.

Mr Smith had watched Mr Jones over the months and sympathized with what he was going through. He knew what it was like to lose a partner but he could not understand why Mr Jones had stopped visiting his wife when she needed him most. For Mr Smith, despite the fact that his wife no longer recognized him and her talk was no longer comprehensible, to be there in the ward at visiting time was what he felt he had to do because he cared.

Is it possible to say which husband cared more for his wife? Did they care equally or was Mr Jones actually doing more even though it seemed that he was doing less? Would our judgement be different if we knew what either wife actually wanted or needed? We do not have to be professional carers to find ourselves making judgements about whether and how people care for one another. And we base our opinions on what we know about ourselves and our relationships with others. We are not afraid to say that caring for a spouse would include continued contact, however distressing for one party. We would put ourselves in the wife's place and we would think of how she would feel, imprisoned in a body that would not work, with a mind that grew tired and with a shattered self-image. We would ask ourselves whether she would want her spouse with her to help her through it and we would conclude that she would. We would argue, as Midgley (1980, p. 340) has, that caring for another person 'means serving their needs as well as wanting to be near them' and is connected 'with thinking highly of them'. In all this we would draw on our ordinary, lay, preprofessional experience.

A capacity for caring is part of human nature. However, to become good at caring one has to make a choice to actualize and develop that capacity (cf. Roach, 1984). In effect, one chooses to work at becoming a certain kind of person.

Two elements in the human capacity for caring are the capacity to *feel* for another person and the capacity to *understand* something of their situation. Positive activities of caring are possible only if one 'tunes in to the same wave length' as the other person. Noddings (1984, p. 16) argues that caring further involves an 'engrossment' or 'motivational displacement' whereby the carer moves away from his or her own viewpoint and looks at things as though from the viewpoint of the other person and makes the other person's motives his or her own.

The universal nature of caring, its reliance on the willingness of the carer to move from self-centredness to other-centredness, and its emphasis on the practicality and wholeness of the relationship are consistent features identified by several writers (Mayeroff, 1971; Heidegger, 1962; Griffin, 1980, 1983).

To care and to be cared for is possible only within a relationship. Being in relationships to other persons (i.e. not isolated or alone) is a basic fact of human existence. Moreover it is good to be in relationship, to be viewed as a human being and to be able to view others as fully integrated persons. In general we do not like being separated from others, particularly those we love; all of us have a natural wish and capacity to be fully integrated with others. We seek integration in our relationships with others through the constant and repeated affirmation of our unique selves and our dependence upon the other person to recognize and cherish that otherness. This process is mutual and in caring relationships is carried on through the openness, receptiveness and authenticity of reactions between the carer and the one being cared for.

Our knowledge of how to care for another person and the desire to do it both come, according to Noddings and others, from our own experiences of being cared for. The composition of our own experiences may equip us more or less effectively to deal with major life experiences. Traditionally, caring has been centred around life events and body practices – puberty, pregnancy, childbirth, care of newborns, care of the sick, old and dying (Colliere, 1986). Before we can engage with someone at one of these life events we must be able to assure the other person of our commitment to act on their behalf, be willing and prepared to sustain continued interest in their experience over time, show a desire to renew the techniques for safe involvement in the relationship (Noddings, 1984, p. 16). The caring relationship assumes the meeting together and the mutual positive regard between the carer and the cared for. This ensures that such factors as maintaining the integrity and dignity of the cared for will be part of caring.

When the balance between motivation, commitment, skills and knowledge and respect for the cared for is distorted a number of potential problems are likely to emerge. Noddings (1984, p. 25) identifies a danger in the caring ceasing to be an activity based on engrossment and motivational displacement and becoming instead an activity of abstract problem-solving. With the latter the focus is not on the person being cared for but on the problem. Then the person entrusted with the caring is taking the objective attitude (see section 1.7, above): while certain requirements for care-taking may be satisfied, the *interpersonal* character of the interactions between the carer and the cared for is missing. When this happens only the illusion of care remains.

It would seem therefore that, far from being a straightforward universal activity occurring in much the way a conditional reflex occurs, caring is vastly more complex and challenging. Equipped with their own life experiences and memories of having been cared for, individuals are constantly being challenged in their relationships to care or not to bother to care. They have a choice, and their choices affect other people in ways which can be labelled either good or bad; this suggests that there is an ethical dimension to the caring relationship.

3.2 THE ETHICAL DIMENSION

What I ought to do for another person and what I actually do may be at variance for a number of reasons. It may not be due to my lack of moral conscience or my lack of concern that someone is not cared for. It may be due to my lack of knowledge or life experience. For example, an experienced ward sister recently recounted the story of how three student nurses reacted to the death of a patient on her ward. They were all in the first year of training, each having the same clinical experience; however, one of the students was a mature married woman with three children while the other two were in their early 20s. The ward sister had noted that while the 'younger students' had stood unsure of themselves and uncertain what to do in the situation, the mature student had immediately responded by taking the grieving relatives into a quiet room and sitting with them, listening and comforting them. This example of a caring response offered by the mature student to the younger nurses reflected her greater life experience. However, given the professional context, it may have intimidated the other students and made them feel guilty about their apparent inability to care.

Feelings of guilt and conflict are at times inescapable consequences of being involved in caring for others, whether in our ordinary lay capacity or as professionals. When we consider what we ought to be doing and how we ought to be caring we are constructing an ethical ideal. Failure to reach that will create its own tensions which will be interpreted as personal failure and culpability, or as a learning experience where the carer is forced to reconsider the components of the particular situation. Conflicts may arise when competing demands for care from several sources render care in the relational sense impossible. It may also occur when what the cared for person wants is not what we think best or when we become overburdened.

It is relatively easy to imagine how, in a situation of conflict and tension, the carer may come to doubt the necessity for caring to be based on a mutual, reciprocal, trusting interaction with the cared for. There is a temptation to reduce caring to a set of services offered to the other person, a collection of actions to be done. But we are prevented from doing this by what Noddings (1987) calls the recognition of our ethical selves. She sees the 'ethical self' as being in an active relation between one's actual self and one's vision of the ideal self as one who is caring and cared for. The ethical self is born of the fundamental recognition of relatedness, that which connects one person to another and which reconnects one through the other back to one's self again. It is the interest in this ethical self that induces the feeling 'I must' and which motivates us to care. Noddings continues:

> At every level in every situation, there are decisions to be made, and we are free to affirm or to reject the impulse to care. But our related-ness, our apprehension of happiness or misery in others, comes through immediately. We may reject what we feel, what we see clearly, but at the risk of separation not only from others but from our ideal selves . . . This linkage, this fundamental relatedness, is at the very heart of our being. Thus I am totally free to reject the impulse to care, but I enslave myself to a particularly unhappy task when I make this choice. I am not naturally alone. I am naturally in a relation . . .
>
> (Noddings, 1984, p. 50)

Each one of us is free to reject the impulse to care, to reduce interactions to the level of abstract problem-solving, to fence off our emotional response to the cared-for, and to assume the objective attitude. This affects us on two levels: the natural level and the ethical level. If we did not want to care and be cared for, if we did not mind suffering and were not liable to despair or if such experiences could not be helped by companionship, then we would not need to put such high value on caring. Nor would it be so impressive to care if it were always easy and pleasant. But we choose what may be distressing to us because we reckon it is worth it. It is good to care, good for the other person, good for ourselves.

With this, an ethical position, as regards caring for others, is beginning to take shape. The basic notions about caring come from our own bio-graphies, our experiences of being cared for. These supply a form that impulses which would otherwise be formless and primitive can take; they can then be recognized as caring impulses. We get a sense of the centrality of the relationship between the carer and the cared for, a relation of mutual acknowledgement between one person and another. Within that relation we find such elements as commitment, trust, friendship, honesty, integrity, faithfulness, compassion, honour, suffering, joy, anger, jealousy and so on. And then we begin to reflect upon our own behaviour and motives and those of the people we care for. Did we really engage with them? Did we really tell the truth? Did they notice how uninterested we were? Perhaps we try to justify ourselves by saying that we cannot be so good all the time. And in thinking this we are recognizing how we are working to some sort of ideal model of how we should be caring. To be the person one wants to be in relation to the well-being of others and to facilitate their good before one's own is a clear declaration of one's ethical position. What motivates us is the desire to care; how we do it is through becoming more like the person we imagine we should be. We constantly check our progress through the interactions with those for whom we care.

The ethics of caring is not to be thought of as mainly a matter of actions which ought to be done; it is to a great extent an ethics of virtue. The foregoing remarks indicate that the maintenance of a caring relationship is dependent upon the carer having developed a number of character traits which could be called virtues, e.g. patience, fortitude, compassion. Here it is important to note that virtues are not bits of baggage that can be selectively taken on board for certain procedures and then discarded. They are attributes which pervade the person's whole life and which have the potential to influence every thought, every decision, every interaction. They unify rather than dissect but they in turn are intelligible only as characteristics 'of a unitary life, a life that can be conceived and evaluated as a whole' (MacIntyre, 1981, p. 191). Whether or not caring itself is a virtue (cf. Noddings, 1984, p. 98), the genuine ethical commitment to maintain one's self as caring gives rise to the development and exercise of virtues. These must be assessed in the context of caring situations.

In the main, little thought is given to such issues by people who care. It is only when problems arise, when conflicts emerge or when responsibilities change that we find ourselves wishing to investigate them more thoroughly. The transition from ordinary carer to professional carer (and particularly nurse) is one period when the individual is confronted by many deep and complex issues. For example, what happens if we find that we cannot care for a particular patient, when our personal reaction is one of distrust, repugnance or hate? Is it acceptable to admit that there will be some people for whom we as human beings cannot care? Or does becoming a professional carer, a nurse, mean that somehow we are expected to develop that extra moral fibre and do the job? Or do we just pretend?

Take student nurse Black's experience. She had just finished her paediatric placement and was looking forward to spending some time in the neonatal unit until she came across Roberta. Roberta was a 15-month, severely deformed hydrocephalic baby who had survived beyond everyone's expectations. Several shunt operations to control the build-up of fluid in her cranium had all been unsuccessful with the result that Roberta's head seemed almost as large as her poorly developed body. Roberta's mother had stopped visiting her a long time ago and no one had ever really been sure about her father. The ward sister in the unit had a special feeling for Roberta and used to go and talk to her, hold her and engage in a range of actions that any mother/carer would do for a normal baby.

Student nurse Black found the whole experience grotesque and was appalled at her own revulsion towards Roberta. Any pity she felt for the child was quickly overtaken by the alarm she experienced in having to go near the child and especially to pick her up. The experience with Roberta challenged her whole notion of herself as a nurse and as a caring person. What ought she to do with the feelings of disgust and revulsion she was experiencing? Should she talk to the ward sister about them? Should she ask for a transfer? Should she pretend she was sick? Should she make sure she would never have to care for Roberta? What nurse Black reckoned to be the problem was the conflict in her own mind between her ideal image of caring for another person and entering into a relationship and the reality of Roberta. The child reminded her not of a human being but of a little monster and thus she found it a struggle to make contact with Roberta in a relational sense.

Her feelings of guilt were accentuated all the more because she could see that the ward sister had been able to 'make contact' with Roberta. She consoled herself by thinking that sister had known her when she had not been so physically distorted, but such thoughts did not extinguish the feelings of failure that she carried round with her. She never did talk to anyone in the unit about her problem.

What is interesting about this example is how student nurse Black perceived her professional duty to care but did not know how to overcome a range of human responses. Often the move from lay carer to nurse or professional carer is a period of extreme challenge to oneself and one's notion of caring.

3.3. THE PROFESSIONALIZATION OF CARE

What the novice brings into nursing in terms of past experiences, character traits and ideal images of caring relationships is quite substantial. Already a self-selection process has been taking place helping the new nurse determine why she wants to become a professional carer. Of course the motives are never totally clear nor are they always altruistic. Yet there has already been established a set of rights and wrongs, dos and don'ts according to the individual's own code of conduct. That such opinions and beliefs are often challenged and contradicted by the reality of professional care is one early problem that nurses have to confront. Melia (1983) illustrates this conflict extremely well in her analysis of the socialization process of the nursing student.

However, she tends to see the components of the ordinary or lay caring relationship as fundamentally different from the professional caring relationship. This difference causes problems for the novice because she is having to change both her understanding of a caring relationship and her views about how it should be conducted.

Melia (1983) sees three important differences between the lay and professional relationships: first, nurses undertake work on a contractual basis rather than on the basis of duty, altruism or necessity; second, nurses and patients are not personally involved in each other's lives, whereas lay-caring usually takes place within the context of a family or friendship; third, the nurse and patient may not have the same outlook, culture, values and expectations whereas the giver and recipient of lay care are likely to have a shared outlook, etc. (Melia, 1983, p. 16).

There is a potential danger in distinguishing the two relationships by reference to the above factors, particularly when implicit in them is the notion that professional care involves the physical and social distancing of the nurse from the patient. If this is what actually happens then the corresponding actions, behaviour and values of the professional carers are ones that belong with an objective attitude rather than a participant attitude. However, the response of many nurses and others (see especially Menzies, 1970) has been to challenge this approach on the grounds of its unacceptability from a human point of view. Also it does not help to explain to the novice whether she is justified in keeping to her lay notion of caring in order not to compromise her more worthy ideals of caring for others. Furthermore, Melia (1983) may be saying that the values of the profession are bound by the impersonality of the professional nursing relationship and that this is the only way that it can be, given the contractual impersonal nature of the relationship.

Another way of looking at the problem of professional values versus individual values is to explore the possibility that professional care is more of an extension or a fulfilment of lay-caring (cf. Kitson, 1987). Then the problem is not one of ensuring an acceptable distance between the nurse and the patient; rather it is about exploring those features of the lay-caring relationship which need enhancement from someone expertly trained in professional care. The natural capacity of the individual to care and their ethical response to the caring relationship are the foundations upon which professional care is built. Rather than distancing themselves from patients, nurses as individuals therefore have to commit themselves to care – to act on behalf of the patient, to continue to be interested in him as a person and continually to renew that commitment, possess a sufficient level of knowledge and skills to ensure that the care being provided is adequate and to make sure that the interaction is built on positive regard and respect for the individuality and integrity of the other person.

The dilemma faced by the student nurse in relation to the distance between herself and the patient has been fuelled as much by the traditional images of nursing as by different ideologies of care. Historically, there has always been confusion over the role of the nurse ranging from nurturer to technical expert. Stinson (1979) has traced the development of the professional nurse from the early folk image of the nurse as a simple mothering care-giver through medieval times where the religious image of the nurse as care-giver for the sick was dominant, to her development as medical technician within an institutional setting. Colliere (1986) is more critical of the social and economic forces which worked on caring over the centuries to change it from an independent therapeutic art centred on body practices and promotion of well-being in the fifteenth and six-teenth centuries to a dependent, devalued activity based upon dedication to the poor and salvation of the soul. This change in orientation paved the way during the nineteenth century for increased value of technical interventions and consideration of care as menial work, worthless, requir-ing no ability, no knowledge, and therefore no economic recognition (cf. Colliere 1986, pp. 99–102).

The continuing tension between performing the tasks of nursing and being a person capable of caring for others has led to much confusion within the profession as to what a good nurse should be like. Colliere (1986, p. 103) illustrates this point by saying that caring is not identified as a specific legitimate and personal activity; rather it was defined in terms of the nurse's role(s) and in terms of specific behaviour attributed to the role(s).

Thus we find a proliferation of roles that the nurse can take on. Curtin *et al.* (1982, p. 86) have summarized a number of them, including physician assistant, caretaker, parent surrogate, champion of the sick, healer, and health educator. Linked to the roles are expectations of the nurse's con-duct. Lamb (1981) found that how the nurse is supposed to behave has changed in nursing accounts from a focus on the moral character traits of the practitioner – unselfish, obedient, tactful, devoted, kind – to an empha-sis on the moral obligation of the nurse in specific circumstances. (See the discussions of virtue and duty in section 2.3 above.) Yet without agreement on whether the nurse is to be acknowledged as a practitioner in her own right by virtue of her distinctive contribution to care, it is difficult to see how a clear picture of what the nurse is expected to do and how the nurse can act intentionally can emerge.

One possible step has been offered by Flaherty, in Curtin and Flaherty (1982, p. 71), who has characterized professional nurses as being educated practitioners, possessing a code of ethics, who are dedicated to the ideal of master craftsmanship in work; who value membership in a professional organization and who are accountable and take responsibility for their own behaviour.

Despite apparent progress on these fronts, nursing has still to resolve the 'distance problem' between its practitioners and the patient. Melia's three categories – the nature of the contractual relationship, the level of intimacy between the professional carer and the patient, and the reciprocity of the relationship in terms of life experiences and values – have rarely been analysed in detail. Instead, there have been, by way of response, exhortations to provide more patient-centred care and to organize nursing according to the individual needs of the patient rather than according to the headings of the medical diagnosis. On their own, such responses may not serve to illuminate caring for nurses, particularly when seen in the light of a history which recommends detachment, distance and devotion.

Our earlier discussion of the nature of the lay-caring relationship (Kitson, 1987) emphasized the fundamental importance of forming the relationship in the first instance, and then sustaining it through continued commitment and regard for the person being cared for. It is only relatively recently that nursing has looked at the nature of the nurse-patient relationship in a way that focused on the individual practitioner taking personal responsibility for the care of a patient (Orlando, 1961; Travelbee, 1971; Kitson, 1987). These findings are interesting in that they show that the nurse–patient relationship was rarely viewed as focused and specific, nor did it carry particular responsibilities and obligations towards one patient. Rather, the commitment of the nurse was to the collective patient population, either in the ward or under the care of a particular consultant. Nurses could be substituted for one another without any problem; what one nurse could do for a group of patients was similar to what any other nurse could do. Such a rationale illustrates how rudimentary the notion of a nurse–patient relationship is and how at odds it is with the whole concept of a caring relationship.

The good news is that, surprisingly perhaps, many professional nurses successfully devise strategies in their practice which help them cope with the paradox of professional care. Yet these practitioners work under the conflict of safeguarding their personal ethical values and notions of intimate caring relationships in the context of what they understand to be professional practice (cf. section 1.6c, above, especially the concluding paragraph). One staff nurse recounts the story of being reprimanded for being too familiar with a patient. The ward sister found her crying with a patient and putting her arm round him to comfort him. Another talked about the displeasure shown toward her by a senior nurse when she explained the reason why she had not finished tidying the ward. It was because she had chosen to spend time helping some students talk through their feelings following the death of a patient. This, according to the senior nurse, was not her main priority.

Rather than deny the contradictions in action and thought that surround professional caring relationships, it would be helpful to explore them more thoroughly and acknowledge their complexity. With the vast body of psychoanalytical and psychotherapeutic literature available to nurses, there is scope for far-reaching exploration of ways to establish, maintain, and terminate relationships with our patients. However, the fundamental problem may not be a lack of understanding of the processes of interaction but more importantly that we are not sure what sort of relationship we want to establish with our patients in the first place.

3.4 THE PROFESSIONALIZATION OF CARING RELATIONSHIPS

Even if we were sure of the sort of relationship that is required, we would then have the problem of equipping practitioners with the right sort of attitudes and skills to be able to care for patients within this model. But in the very act of professionalizing an activity, one runs the risk of distorting it. Rhodes (1986) illustrates this phenomenon within social work as related to case work practice. The working assumption here is that certain people could and should be helped through the medium of interpersonal relationships; and it is part of the skill and professional responsibility of the helping persons to know what the components of a helpful relationship are and to incorporate them consciously, in so far as that is possible, into their dealings with people. Such personal qualities as warmth, acceptance, empathy, concern and genuineness are seen as central to the relationship.

Yet Rhodes (1986, p. 163) goes on to explore how the structure of the worker – client relationship can undermine the very qualities it is meant to establish. Looking at the comments from satisfied clients one is struck by clients' perception of the good social worker as being more of a friend than a professional. The client's satisfaction and change in circumstances were dependent on their perception of the workers as friends. Such friendships had the following qualities – empathy, caring, flexibility, patience, suggestions rather than advice, reciprocity in the form of the sharing of one's personal life and provision of immediate concrete help in the mode requested. Sainsbury (1974) also found that clients put high priority on social workers' moral goodness and ethical integrity. Her studies revealed that for casework to be effective workers had to act like friends, conveying not only warmth, acceptance, empathy, but also some reciprocity in sharing, concrete help, social activities, and respect for the relationship as an end in itself. The social worker was required to be willing to disclose herself in particular ways and involve herself within the relationship.

There is always the tension between seeming to become too involved, and therefore unable to be objective, and being too detached. One common factor identified by Rhodes (1986, p. 85) within social work practice, but which is pertinent to nursing, is how the language used can serve to disguise our moral judgements by making us experts and by making clients into medical entities, or by making procedures and goals seemingly value free. The danger Rhodes envisages with this, is that by distancing us from clients and describing issues as technical, our language encourages us to disrespect our clients in subtle ways – they quite easily can be relegated to the status of 'cases to be handled' through professional training (cf. section 1.7, above). Melia (1983) discussed this problem in terms of labelling patients and marginalizing certain difficult or unpopular patients through social sanctions.

A final question is how far a personal concern for someone is compatible with the intention of changing them or their behaviour. In the social work context Sainsbury (1974) asks whether, if one's chief goal is developing the relationship, one is not acting professionally to bring about a specifiable change. If, however, one's chief goal is to change the person, then surely the personal concern will be manipulative. Sainsbury (1974) concludes that this sort of caring is an odd sort; it is not genuine in the sense of being for its own sake but is created only in order to accomplish some other purpose. This last comment is relevant to the nursing situation. Can a caring relationship be established between a nurse and a patient solely in order to accomplish the medical or nursing goals of recovery? Must there be some sort of reciprocal pay-off between the nurse and the patient for the relationship to be of mutual benefit and therefore a caring one? Are there distinctive patient goals which can be achieved only within the well-defined parameters of a nurse–patient relationship? Is this what we want and does it conform to our best image of what a caring relationship between the nurse and the patient should be like?

Professionalizing any caring relationship, be it nursing or social work, brings its own set of problems. These are related not only to the socialization process and professional values that have built up over the years but also to a number of inherent paradoxes in attempting to professionalize care (see Campbell, 1984a, for a fuller analysis of this). What is central to the argument is what we use as our image of how it should be done. And we must not permit the apparent rigidity of a professional system to carry more weight in our thinking than our own experiences of caring and being cared for. Thus, the ethical dilemmas described by Melia (1983) as resulting from the tension between the student nurse's lay conception of caring and professional care should continue for as long as the actions of the professional compromise deeper, more lasting, impressions of what caring really ought to be like. To test this statement we must explore what sort of person a professional carer would be and what sort of relationship they would construct with their patients.

3.5 CHARACTERISTICS OF THE PROFESSIONAL CARER AND THE CARING RELATIONSHIP

Early writers on ethics for nurses stressed obedience to the physician as one of the most important characteristics of the professional nurse. She must become a faithful servant to her master (Moore, 1945, p. 38), while for Dock (1917) obedience was the very cornerstone of good nursing. Failure to be obedient was seen as the first stumbling block for beginners and it was only when the nurse could obey without question that she would ever be seen as reliable.

Linked with the virtue of obedience was the notion that nursing was essentially a vocation. Osler (quoted in Pearce, 1969) describes nursing as one of the highest callings in life, saying that in nursing

> a woman may not reach the ideals of her soul, she may fall short of the ideals of her head, but she will go far to satiate the longings of the heart from which no woman can escape.

This curious concentration on ideals (which the nurse may well fall short of) may have its roots in the religious influences affecting the development of nursing and caring for the sick. However that may be, it is interesting that no other professional caring group has so much devotion, so much dedication and so much mission expected of it. Whilst the concepts of devotion and commitment have been used to describe the level of engagement needed by other professional groups to respond effectively to patients and clients (cf. e.g. Mayeroff, 1971; Noddings, 1984; Campbell, 1984a), none of these newer professional groups chooses to relate such personal traits to solely moral virtues.

In other words, in those other groups devotion is seen as part of the range of attributes necessary to do the job: the inference is that the practitioner chooses to develop it, or recognizes the fact that she or he has to pay attention to nurturing it. In contrast, the implicit assumption running through nursing texts is that the nurse is already devoted, is compassionate and has a sense of mission in order to select the job in the first place. Such notions have at least two effects; first, they place unrealistic expectations upon new nurses to be 'perfect' nurses as well as near-perfect people, and second, they deny the possibility of nurses ever being able, or needing, to learn how to be more devoted, more committed, more compassionate towards their patients.

The psychotherapeutic literature and concepts such as Rogers' (1961) therapeutic-use-of-the-self within clearly defined relationships have helped to describe more clearly those general characteristics of people involved in caring for others. The freedom to discuss how one uses one's own personality and presence as a way of influencing and directing the experience and well-being of another person has begun to put into words and concepts those encounters nurses and other carers knew were important.

But why should we be bothered to use ourselves in a therapeutic way? In beginning to think about this we may find ourselves back with Noddings' image of the ideal self and one's best memory of caring and being cared for which we recognized as an ethical stance. Perhaps we choose to develop our interpersonal and caring skills because we have a desire to meet the ethical demands of our image of caring and being cared for. This need not mean being branded from the start as obedient, devoted, dedicated people with a vocation. We may concentrate instead on those characteristics described by Mayeroff (1971) as epitomizing any caring relationship. We want to acquire the right knowledge, the proper sensitivity to atmosphere and interactions, an adequate measure of patience and honesty. We desire the ability to trust the potential in others to enable them to grow in their own way. We wish to have the humility to constantly seek to learn about others, never to give up hope and always to have enough courage to be able to take risks which are calculated according to one's past and present experiences and one's knowledge of the best good for the other person. We want to be free to admit that we do not know how to do all these things but we do want to learn.

Noddings emphasizes the need for the carer to become engrossed in the other person's experience and to be able to step back from their own desires. This reflects the main items identified in Mayeroff's (1971) list. Similarly, Rhodes' (1986) set of attributes seen as essential for a good social worker includes compassion, warmth, honesty, moral courage, hopefulness, humility, acceptance, genuineness, and authenticity.

The extra dimension added to the above lists by nursing authors relates to the physical intimacy between the nurse and the person being cared for. Perhaps it is because of this 'bodily presence' (Campbell, 1984, p. 50) that nursing has chosen to retain a number of more puritanical notions about the nature of the nurse's therapeutic-use-of-self. Indeed, it is only relatively recently that techniques such as massage, reflexology, and aromatherapy have been accepted as legitimate nursing practice. The final recognition that the nurse touches the patient in a positive therapeutic way (cf. Colliere, 1986, pp. 97, 100) has interesting implications for all the other times the nurse touches the patient – during dressing, washing, going to the toilet, bathing, feeding and so on. And if nursing interventions are seen as therapeutic because of the presence of the nurse, then all the nurse's interventions are potentially therapeutic.

In terms of characteristics, therefore, one expects the nurse to be able to handle the body of the other person in a way that overcomes embarrassment and leaves a sense of privacy intact (Campbell, 1984a, p. 50). This aspect of practical care is about demonstrating kindness, concern, sensitivity, and using the physical closeness of bodies to a therapeutic end, overcoming weakness and restoring hope.

3.6 EQUAL CARE FOR EACH?

Yet the access the nurse has to the body and mind of another person places both her and the patient in a potentially hazardous position, particularly when one recalls the problems related to professional caring. In the context of casework practice, Sainsbury (1974) noted that clients found the most effective social workers to be those who treated them as friends and who disclosed information about themselves. If we extend this finding to professional nursing practice we could say that the best nurses are those who are perceived as friends. Indeed Campbell (1984) describes nurses as companions to the sick. However, it is only in the most intimate of relationships that we would ever expose our bodies and minds to another person. It would only be in situations where trust and fidelity were guaranteed, where integrity and confidentiality were also assumed (see Chapter Six below).

How then can the nurse guarantee this sort of fidelity and trust when she cares for a range of individuals? Either she takes the relationship seriously and constructs the proper qualities around it which lead it on in a therapeutic way, bathed in trust and comfort that both parties are giving and receiving from one another, or else she risks engaging only superficially, immersed as she is in the dos and don'ts of professional practice. That the nurse has had to confront issues related to being honest, open, concerned, authentic, compassionate, courageous, patient, responsive, and sensitive is implied in the very suggestion that she has to choose between being involved with her patients and being detached from them. Even if she chooses to be involved with some and detached from others, she has exercised a choice the consequence of which will provide one sort of caring relationship to one patient and another sort to a different patient.

That there is always a choice to make does not in itself mean that the nurse is going to fail if she does not lavish the same amount of 'tender loving care' upon every patient. A fundamental premise of any caring relationship is that it is reciprocal in nature (Noddings, 1984; Buber, 1958). Something from the carer must be received and completed in the recipient of that care. Noddings (1984) implies that this something is generally characterized as an attitude – the cared-for is looking for something which tells him the carer has regard for him. It is, to use Marcel's word, a certain 'disposability' or readiness to bestow and spend one's self and make one's self available (cf. Blackham, 1959, p. 80). If the cared-for is with someone who makes themselves indisposable, Marcel describes the response in the cared-for as being made to feel as if he does not exist, he is thrown back on to and into himself. Both parties know when this happens but, according to Noddings (1984), it is the responsibility of the one caring to find a solution.

However, the recipient of care has a part to play in the relationship. Among other things, he must be willing to respond to the one caring and to continue to disclose information about himself and how he wants to be helped. If this is not possible then the carer is faced with working in a relationship where the expenditure of themselves is not reflected in the other person. Perhaps the real test of a caring relationship is where the commitment, engrossment and motivational displacement of the carer are neither recognized nor desired by the recipient of the care. Certainly, the most challenging nurse–patient relationships are those where the patient either rejects the support offered or is incapable – through disability, illness or mental state – of responding to the carer. The question arising from such situations relates to whether it is possible to care for another person when natural affection and receptivity break down. Do professional carers move from a natural responsiveness to an ethical responsibility to provide care in spite of the non-response from the other person? Or is it impossible to provide care when one party is unwilling or unable to respond as a human being? The problem is that the demands of the professional caring role exclude full-blown participant attitude responses (such as indignation or huffiness) to such unresponsiveness. There may be possibilities of maintaining a personal caring relationship in an 'as if' way while making use of the objective attitude as a resource from time to time as the occasion demands (cf. Strawson, 1982, p. 67, and section 1.7, above). One possibility is to adopt the objective attitude permanently and offer gardener-solicitude (cf. Dennett, 1982, p. 158, and sections 1.7 and 2.5, above) in place of full personal care. (The suitability of this as a last resort in the case of a recalcitrantly unresponsive patient does not mean that the objective attitude should characterize ordinary nurse–patient interactions.)

It is important to remind ourselves that just as the carers will have choices to make about how they care, so too will the recipients of care have decisions to make regarding the nature of the relationship. If the person receiving care experiences a sense of isolation and rejection, he may still choose by an act of ethical heroism (Noddings, 1984, p.78) to respond and thus contribute to the caring relationship. Thus the cared-for can act as the guide and support for the carer. This situation gives weight to the possibility that one can learn both to care and to be cared for. (Perhaps everyone in society should receive training for being recipients of care.) Again, that either party is exercising a choice in how they are to establish and maintain the relationship reflects the possibility of their working to an ideal image of what it should be like.

3.7 WHO NEEDS PROFESSIONAL CARE?

An important question is how individuals know they need to seek help from professional carers and particularly from nurses. We have been making a number of assumptions about the client's ability to recognize their need for care and the nurse's willingness and competence to meet that need. Even though such questions belong more to the domain of nursing theory than nursing ethics, it is important to establish a number of common principles.

First, from a traditional medical model, one can argue that the individual recognizes his need for nursing care as secondary to his detecting some dysfunction or discomfort preventing him from undertaking his daily activities of living. Fitzpatrick (1984) outlines the complex factors that influence the individual's assessment of his need for medical help, identifying cultural, social, economic and psychological factors as impinging upon the final judgement. Whilst the doctor commonly will see the individual case as a presentation of symptoms reflecting an underlying disease (Stinson and Webb, 1975), the patient (because that is what he is fast becoming) presents problems and rationales for why and how those problems might exist. Stinson and Webb (1975) suggest there is almost a ritual order governing the form in which problems are actually presented, priority being given to physical symptoms with fears and anxieties about possible reasons for the illness being left until the end to be discussed. It is almost as if the doctor is dealing with two separate but interrelated issues; one is the clinical signs and symptoms being presented before him and the other is the perceptions and concerns that organize and motivate the patient's consultation.

Second, the most common way for the nurse to engage with the patient is following – or as a result of – the person's decision to seek medical assistance. This may be in the context of the community, where the general practitioner requests that one of the health care team visit the patient either to undertake a specifically medically determined task or (preferably) to undertake their own nursing assessment. Our more common perception, however, is of the interdependence between doctor and nurse in the institutional setting where the medical decision for treatment necessitates a number of reactions and interventions on the part of the nurse.

These two factors often mask the third principle which has to do with the independent and often quite distinct nature of the person's potential need for care from a nurse as opposed to care from a doctor. Medical conditions as presented and perceived by the individual are not only formal clinical manifestations of disease. They are also affected by lay concepts of illness and the derivation of those illnesses (see Sontag, 1978 for an interesting discussion of the way society perceives TB and cancer).

While the doctor's primary concern is the treatment of the disease, it is often left to the observations of the nurse to help the individual make sense of the events he has now become party to.

Of course, the preferred situation is that both doctor and nurse assist the person to construct a meaning to his experience of illness. But this would require the establishment and maintenance of effective communication channels between both parties. Traditionally, the doctor–patient relationship has contained more boundaries and roles (Chapters Four and Five, below) which determine the limits of behaviour and obligations of either party. What we are arguing in this chapter is that the nurse–patient relationship requires a similar set of parameters to be identified in order for the patient to obtain the best results from his interaction with the nurse.

The nurse–patient relationship, it is proposed, is based on an understanding of the complex dynamics that naturally occur between two people who care for each other. Built on to these foundations is the nurse's ability to identify those needs, most commonly derived from the person's experience of illness or disability, which constitute nursing needs. Such nursing needs arise for three major reasons (cf. Kitson, 1987).

First, they can emerge because the lay carer (spouse, friend, parent, relative or the person himself or herself) no longer has the knowledge or skill to maintain the individual at an acceptable level of functioning. For example, an elderly person living alone and being cared for by her daughter, falls and fractures her hip. The competence of the daughter to deal with this situation is limited, particularly in the acute phase of the illness but even in the recovery and rehabilitation stage.

Secondly, nursing needs can arise because of the potential lay carer's lack of commitment. Suppose the elderly lady's daughter, having admitted her mother to hospital, then decides that she does not want to look after her or help her return home. This lack of commitment to care would be another reason why professional nursing interventions would be required. One can imagine that in such situations the nurse would be concerned not only with the patient's physical and functional recovery but also with helping her to work through her feelings of rejection and anger and perhaps even diminution of the will to go on living produced by her daughter's rejection of her.

Thirdly, planned nursing intervention is needed in cases in which the carer, for any one of a number of reasons, begins to treat the cared-for as an object rather than respecting them as human beings. The strain on some individuals caring continuously for their dependent relatives cannot be overestimated and often the professional intervention comes at a time of severe strain on the whole caring network. The nurse's job is to intervene to protect the vulnerable individual but also to try and preserve and foster any reciprocity that may be left between the carer and the cared for. It may be that the nurse finds herself negotiating not only with the patient but also with a number of individuals in the wider caring context in order to re-establish an acceptable caring relationship that will maintain the needs of all parties.

For relationships of this sort to be established it is essential that the nurse have a sense of her clinical role as well as a thorough understanding of the dimensions and boundaries of her interpersonal role. The latter role is established on partnership and on a set of principles which acknowledge the distinct service nursing offers to society. The ultimate goal of the nurse–patient relationship is to seek to promote optimum independence in the patient so that the patient can be maintained within normal lay caring relationships or, failing this, so that the professional caring relationship can create the conditions for the cared-for to flourish without adverse effects to their self-esteem or personal identity.

3.8 CONCLUSION

The path toward becoming a professional carer is both complex and challenging. There is the need to develop one's own notions of caring and being cared for as remembered and to reflect these experiences against one's idea of the ideal self and the ideal caring relationship. The commitment required to enter into such an inquiry is considerable, as it has the potential to challenge every relationship one has experienced and will possibly make one more conscious of one's motives and methods of interaction in future relationships. However, such risk-taking is necessary as it frees the individual sufficiently to help him prepare to become involved in the experience of others, not just as an objective spectator but as an actor on the stage of another person's life story. The ability to be involved in an unselfish or altruistic way is possible through the motivational displacement necessary to enter into a caring relationship. Such displacement must be accompanied by a truthfulness and authenticity of word and action which involve disclosing one's self in particular ways and involving one's self with a particular demeanour in a relationship.

A range of attributes has been identified by writers on the subject of helping relationships. These are the characteristics which are to be nurtured in the carer. They are not assumed to be there already. Rather, the carer is encouraged to reflect upon their own moral development within the context of the caring relationship. Thus the analysis of how one is and how one behaves within the relationship takes on as much importance as the need to develop the proper skills, knowledge and expertise to perform certain tasks within the relationship.

Little has been said about the relationship between the carer and the wider circle of family and friends related to the primary recipient of care. This is a subject that will be discussed more fully in the next chapter. What we have concentrated on here is a discussion of how our natural capacity of caring is extended and influenced by making it a professional activity. We see the guiding light in both situations as the individual's perception of their ideal or ethical selves in relation. We must also note that this picture is a highly fragile and sensitive one in that by our very analysis of it we run the risk of petrifying it and thereby robbing it of the vitality and spontaneity necessary to sustain it. But in discovering these things about caring relationships we draw closer to understanding how we should be and what we want to become in order to care. That our discussions have led us through several lists of personal qualities often described as virtues, e.g. honesty, integrity, truthfulness, fidelity, genuineness, etc., should be no surprise because we started with the notion that caring relationships are based on our desire to provide what is good for another person. Our own ethical dilemmas come when we begin to unpack some of the paradoxes in ordinary caring and professional care, in traditional and realistic images of nursing and in the choices we as individuals are constantly making between involvement and detachment, therapeutic-use-of-self and self-protection, between authenticity and manipulation in every caring relationship we experience.

FOUR

Who is in charge?

4.1 INTRODUCTION

Our perspective on the nature of the relationship between the nurse and the patient, built up in the previous chapter, is founded firmly on the notion of a reciprocal caring relationship. In Chapter Three we proposed that the obligations the nurse has to the patient presuppose a personal relationship, willingly entered into, that calls forth her capacity to care, that requires a level of concern for the other person and a moving away from an exclusive concern with her own best interests to respond to the needs of another person. This is possible only through the meeting together of two individuals, where the interaction is based on mutual respect, positive regard, trust and fidelity.

Such an interpretation assumes a number of things about the nature of the relationship. First, it assumes that both parties are free to engage with each other and that they can terminate the relationship when they choose. It also presupposes a level of equality between the carer (nurse) and one cared for (patient). The carer is refraining from exerting her power over the cared-for because the relationship is based on partnership and on the continual offering of support and help by the carer to the cared-for in order to restore the cared-for's sense of self.

This attractive – if rather idealized – picture of the caring relationship raises a number of questions. For example, what happens to the caring relationship if the patient does not want to accept the care being offered by the nurse? Is the patient free to reject a relationship that is regarded as beneficial to their welfare and which would hasten their recovery? When the patient or one being cared for is incapacitated and a relationship based on partnership or mutual positive regard is impossible to establish, what sort of nurse–patient relationship is possible? When the two parties in a caring relationship are unequal, how does the nurse make decisions about the best interest of the patient? Is it acceptable for her to decide on the patient's behalf because she has got to know him and could predict what sort of decision he would make if he were able to?

Furthermore, the nurse–patient relationship rarely exists in isolation. It is meshed in a complex web of other professional and lay caring relationships, some of which are perceived as more important, some as less important. How does the rhetoric of the caring relationship stand up against more traditional professional relationships such as that between the doctor and the patient? What tensions are created within the lay caring relationship as a result of the patient's need for professional help? And how are these issues related to the nurse's desire to care for the patient in a therapeutic way?

The above questions relate to the fundamental ethical principles of beneficence and autonomy (cf. section 2.4, above) and to the problem of paternalism. Doing one's best for the patient and particularly ensuring that no harm comes to them is the essence of the beneficence model of health care. Yet this beginning point assumes that the professional is always in an advantageous position to the patient, having the knowledge, skill, competence and ability to meet the needs of the other person. Given this imbalance, the only sensible role for the patient is to do what he is told.

Overriding the wishes of the patient or not considering them in a serious way is an extreme form of paternalism, whereby the professional's sense of what is best for the patient (from a medical or nursing point of view) overrides the patient's own self-determination and right to decide. The principle of autonomy is one which presents the importance of the individual's right to make his own decisions about his life and be responsible for the consequences.

At first glance it would seem that by adopting the egalitarian caring model based on a partnership between the nurse and the patient, we are circumventing these bigger issues. By advocating an open, mutually respectful relationship based on engrossment and motivational displacement (Noddings, 1984, p. 16) the nurse will avoid running into the same dilemmas as her medical colleagues in particular, when it comes to deciding what is best for the patient. But is this the case?

4.2 MR D'S PACEMAKER

Consider the following case:

During a post-clinical conference, a . . . nursing student described her dilemma . . . 'when I first began to work with Mr D., I discovered that his pacemaker was no longer working, but that he did not want to have it replaced. I decided that one of my goals would be to convince him that he should replace the pacemaker. But now I wonder if I'm right. He tells me that he is an old man, 84, and that since his wife died he is just 'existing' here in the nursing home, with nothing to live for. He can't see why he should prolong his life by having another pacemaker put in. Doesn't he have the right to make that decision?'

(Ryden, 1978, p. 705)

Ryden (1978) reports that the student's dilemma created an interesting discussion of the patient's rights and responsibilities (his right to autonomy) as well as the role of the nurse and her obligation to provide the best care (principle of beneficence) within the context of a nurse–patient relationship based on partnership in care and mutuality. As the discussion progressed, conflicting values began to emerge and to be compared as to their order of priority in determining what was the right thing to do. Was the maintenance of life itself the most important value regardless of patient circumstances, or was it the quality of life? And what about the autonomy of the individual? Was it possible to extrapolate from the facts and assess the consequences of different actions and weigh up the benefits and risks? And, finally, whose decision was it when it was finally made? Did the nurse make it on behalf of Mr D or was the nurse's problem how best to help him in his decision-making? What if Mr D was found to be suffering from depression following his wife's death? Did this make him incapable of making a rational decision about his own welfare? Even though he voiced an opinion, perhaps it could be disregarded on the ground that he was incompetent in the area of decision-making and this it was acceptable, indeed necessary, for the nurse to make the decision for him.

What are the underlying ethical principles that the nurse would have to consider before she could decide what was the best thing to do for Mr D?

4.3 THE PATIENT AUTONOMY MODEL

Autonomy is self-determination; it is the ability to understand one's situation, to deliberate, to make plans and choices, and to pursue personal goals. The principle of autonomy affirms the individual's sovereignty over her or his own life (cf. section 2.4, above). According to the principle of autonomy, the values and choices of the individual are to be major considerations in any other party's deliberation about matters mainly concerning that individual, whether the other person be a doctor, nurse or friend. If the individual's personal values (cf. section 2.3b, above) conflict with those of the other party, a fundamental responsibility of that party

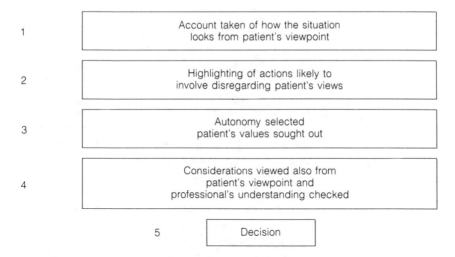

Figure 4.3 Deliberation shaped by the patient autonomy model.

is to respect and facilitate the person's self-determination in making decisions.

The principle of autonomy is central to what we shall call **the patient autonomy model**. This is a way of thinking about patients, about situations involving patients, and about the relationships between patients and health professionals. It involves a collection of shared assumptions, dispositions and expectations. As far as deliberation is concerned, it is a way of appreciating situations and identifying practical options and appraising those options. To the extent that moral deliberation is influenced by the patient autonomy model, its situation-appreciations will give prominence to those features of a situation that can be seen as making contact with the autonomy principle, the autonomy principle will be selected whenever there is any scope for its application, reasons for action backed by that principle will be regarded as more weighty than other reasons for action, and actions supported by those reasons will be more likely to be decided upon (Figure 4.3).

Suppose the question to be answered concerns the sort of care or treatment a patient is to receive. Stage 1 of the health professional's deliberation is her appreciation of the situation. The professional will note the main features of the situation, how it has arisen, and what can be expected to happen later. She will also try to take account of how the situation looks from the viewpoint of the patient. She will be aware of the possibility that grasping this cannot be done in one go, and she will be alert for signs that she has missed some factor that matters to the patient.

At stage 2 she reviews the possible courses of action that could be taken. If a course of action would involve disregarding the patient's own plans or views about what is important in his life, this will be highlighted in the stage 2 review; it will not go unnoticed or be viewed as marginal.

At stage 3 the autonomy principle will be selected, as will any other principles (such as the veracity principle or confidentiality principle) which can be connected with the situation or the possible courses of action. But, as well as making selections from her own personal and professional principles and values, the deliberating professional will actively seek out such of the patient's values and considered preferences and conception of how to live as bear upon the situation or the options.

Then, when it comes to stage 4 and the identifying and weighing of considerations relating to the particular situation, she will be noting considerations not only from her own viewpoint but also as though from the viewpoint of the patient. As far as possible she will continually test her understanding of that viewpoint by putting it into words so that the patient has a chance to put right any misapprehensions. At stage 4 the fact that a course of action would involve overriding the patient's values (a fact that will have been already salient at stage 2) will count heavily as a reason for not taking that course of action.

Finally, at stage 5, the professional will arrive at a conclusion as to what course of action is to be taken in the light of all the stage 4 considerations. To the extent that time permits, though, the outcome of stage 5 and each other stage can be tentative; earlier stages can be returned to and reconsidered in the light of tentative outcomes of later stages.

An autonomous person can deliberate and act (cf. Beauchamp and Childress, 1983, p. 56). Respecting the autonomy of another person involves not dictating what that person should believe or do. The patient autonomy model highlights whatever scope there is for regarding each person as free to choose how they want to live and what values they live by. But are all people capable of acting autonomously? Should everyone be allowed to decide things for themselves? We can immediately think of groups of people whom we could classify as incapable or incompetent to deliberate, choose, and act according to their choices in a rational and balanced manner. Moreover, an individual will typically have different levels of autonomy at different times and at different developmental stages. We return to this problem area below.

4.4 MEDICAL BENEFICENCE, NURSING AUTONOMY

Recognition of and respect for a patient's autonomy are not easily traceable in the classical medical ethics texts that rather stress beneficence and paternalism (cf. Beauchamp and McCullough, 1984, p. 44); and whilst professional codes have looked at principles such as nonmaleficence (doing no harm – cf. section 2.4, above) and beneficence they have said little about veracity, autonomy and justice (cf. Beauchamp and Childress, 1983, p. 11). On the other hand, some groups – eg the American Hospital Association, the Community Health Council and NAWCH – have formulated statements of patients' rights that invoke such principles as autonomy and veracity.

Patients' rights, the right of self-determination, rights to a certain standard of care and rights in care feature increasingly in nurses' discussions of ethical issues related to caring for patients. Unlike the medical codes of conduct, a nursing code such as the *ICN Code for Nurses* (ICN, 1973) makes explicit the nurse's acknowledgement of the 'respect for life, dignity and rights of man'. It goes on to state that the 'nurse, in providing care, promotes an environment in which the values, customs and spiritual beliefs of the individual are respected'; Curtin and Flaherty (1982, p. 9) also argue for a human or patients' rights perspective in outlining the relationship between the patient and the nurse. They connect the individual's right to health care (and nursing) with society's responsibility to recognize basic human needs as related to the promotion of health and prevention of illness. A similar argument has been advanced in a document published by the RCN (1987) entitled 'In Pursuit of Excellence' where the provision of a nursing service to society was seen to be based on the individual's right to expect a level of care and the nurse's professional obligation to provide it.

In considering the autonomous actions of others it is vital that we respect them as persons with the same right to their choice and actions as we have to ours. Thus the rightful respect required by any person is to be given for no other reason than that another individual is a person and rightfully determines their own destiny. Respecting another person's autonomy requires that the person be enabled to order their values and beliefs and to choose and act free from the controlling interventions of others. We have already identified potential problems about this, related to the fact that there are some people who cannot make autonomous decisions and others are not permitted to make them. What is important in considering the principle of autonomy as it relates to medical and nursing care is how one controls the biases derived from the professional perspectives which are constructed from a different knowledge and power base and quite often from a different set of values and beliefs about such central issues as life, death, pain, suffering, and so on.

This is illustrated by a study carried out by McNeil *et al.* (1981) of preferences concerning treatment for cancer of the larynx. McNeil's (1981) study looked at how people view the trade-off between quantity and quality of life in the face of making a decision between a laryngectomy (removal of the larynx) and radiation therapy for the treatment of cancer. What the study showed was that a significant proportion of subjects were more likely to select the radiation therapy even though it offered a decreased chance of survival. What they focused on was the quality of life benefits they gained, by keeping their larynx intact and by not having to undergo surgery. The ethical conclusion to be drawn from this study is that it is not enough simply to present a patient with quantitative aspects of prognosis, e.g. percentage survival after a certain period of time. The way patients assign values to these quantitative outcomes must be considered and respected. On matters of value, the doctor may not know best.

Let us return now to the case set out in section 4.2. At stage 4 of her deliberation, the student nurse had noted the patient's right to decide what to do about his own pacemaker and had noted also the value to be secured by having the pacemaker replaced. The patient's right to decide and the requirements of the nurse's professional concept of the mutuality within the nurse–patient relationship were reasons for her to take the option of letting the patient decide. The benefit of having the pacemaker replaced was a reason to try to get that done. In discussing the case with her classmates, moreover, the student nurse became aware that her own preprofessional values and beliefs also entered into her thinking. She felt she could not stand by and agree to do nothing for Mr D if any harm would come to him as a result. The question was whether she would be acting paternalistically – or maternalistically (Taylor *et al.*, 1989) – if she were to persuade Mr D to do something different. Was his decision really an autonomous one? And, from her own professional perspective, how could she be sure that her lack of action was not a betrayal, a failure to do her best for the patient?

4.5 THE BENEFICENCE MODEL

In general we have moral reason to treat persons as autonomous. We also have reason act beneficently, that is to 'contribute to their welfare, including their health' (Beauchamp and Childress, 1983, p. 148; cf. section 2.4, above). Beneficence has two main aspects; namely, providing positive benefits and producing an optimum balance of benefits over harms (in particular harms that might be related to the treatment or procedure). Many of the professional codes of conduct include statements regarding the knowledge, skills and diligence that practitioners require to execute their professional role in a way that will cause no harm. Some commentators view the 'do no harm' or nonmaleficence principle as more important than the beneficence principle. Accordingly they especially stress the importance of taking full account not only of probable benefit but also of risks and any harm occurring at the time of a procedure or treatment.

The promotion of the patient's good, as perceived and defined by the medical profession, and the avoidance of harms, as the profession sees those harms, are the key aspects of the beneficence model (described in Chapter Two of Beauchamp and McCullough, 1984). With the beneficence model, not only the failure to avoid harm but also the failure to benefit others when in a position to do so violates professional duty. The model also offers a view of the professional–patient relationship, where the patient's best interests are understood exclusively from the viewpoint of medicine; i.e. the body of 'tested knowledge, skills and experience constituting the science and art of the care, alleviation and prevention of disease and injury' (Beauchamp and McCullough, 1984, p. 22). The beneficence model thus provides an objective view of the patient's best interests, the goals of medicine being understood in terms of goods to be sought for patients and harms to be avoided. The principles of nonmaleficence and beneficence themselves are extremely general. They are given more specific content in the context of the medical profession by a long tradition that includes the duty of the doctor to cure disease and injury if there is reasonable hope, and the duty to avoid, prevent or remove specific kinds of harm, namely the pain and suffering of injury and disease (see Beauchamp and McCullough, 1984, p. 30).

A person whose deliberation is influenced by the model will tend to be guided especially by the beneficence and nonmaleficence principles, thus giving greatest weight to patients' welfare as they see it; and they will see situations correspondingly, so that welfare-relevant factors will be salient in their situation-appreciations. Welfare will be seen in terms of the specific kinds of harm and benefit built in to the model.

We see, then, that the medical beneficence model involves some background factors that a deliberating professional will bring to the situation. These include the principles of nonmaleficence and beneficence, specifically medical interpretations of the general evaluative notions of good and harm, and an interpretation of professionals' responsibilities in value terms; i.e. as responsibilities to bring about medical goods and to prevent, remove or ameliorate medical harms (cf. Beauchamp and McCullough, 1984, p. 30).

These background factors will significantly influence the course of deliberation. Along with the non-maleficence and beneficence principles comes a tendency for these principles to be more readily selected at stage 3 than other principles and a tendency for stage 4 considerations based on these principles to have more weight than other stage 4 considerations. Given the specifically medical interpretations of value notions, good will be seen in terms of health and prolonged life, and harm be seen in terms of illness,

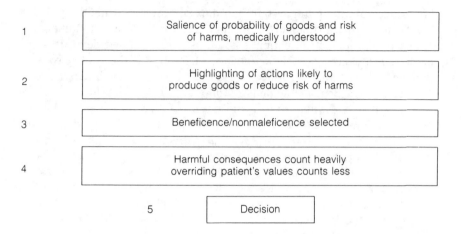

Figure 4.5 Deliberation shaped by the medical beneficence model.

disease, injury, unnecessary pain and suffering, handicapping conditions and premature death (see Beauchamp and McCullough, 1984, pp. 30, 32). Aspects of the situation or the consequence of possible courses of action that can be brought under these headings will be salient in the stage 1 appreciation and in the stage 2 review of possible courses of action. In view of the interpretation of professional responsibilities in value terms, some of the value considerations entering into stage 4 will be reinforced by duty considerations: that a certain course of action will cause medical harm is a reason not to take it; that the professional has a special responsibility not to bring about harm of that kind is an additional reason for the professional not to take that course of action (see Figure 4.5).

Suppose, as before, that a professional has to consider the sort of care or treatment a patient is to receive. Stage 1 of the health professional's deliberation is her appreciation of the situation. The professional will note the main features of the situation, how it has arisen, and what can be expected to happen later. She will be especially sensitive to ways in which what can be expected to happen later includes goods and harms to the patient or the probability of goods and the risk of harms. Here goods and harms will be understood in the medical way.

At stage 2 she reviews the possible courses of action that could be taken. She will note especially that some courses of action improve the probability of goods or reduce the risk of harms to come. These aspects of possible courses of action will be highlighted in the stage 2 review. The fact that a possible course of action fits badly with the patient's personal plans may go unnoticed or be viewed as marginal.

At stage 3 the nonmaleficence and beneficence principles will be selected. Medically interpreted value headings will also be selected where they can be seen to connect with the situation or possible courses of action.

Then, when it comes to stage 4 and the identifying and weighting of considerations relating to the particular situation, she will be endeavouring to maintain an objective attitude and to take account only of value and other considerations that are impersonal. The fact that a course of action is likely to have harmful consequences (a fact that will have been already salient at stage 2) will count heavily as a reason for not taking that course of action. On the other hand, the fact that a course of action would involve overriding the patient's values may well not have been salient at stage 2 and will be a less weighty reason for not taking that course of action.

Finally, at stage 5, the professional will arrive at a conclusion as to what course of action is to be taken in the light of all the stage 4 considerations. To the extent that time permits, though, the outcome of stage 5 and each other stage can be tentative, as before; earlier stages can be returned to and reconsidered in the light of tentative outcomes of later stages.

4.6 CONFLICTS ABOUT THE PATIENT'S GOOD

Often conflicts arise between nursing and medical staff over what should be done for the patient, not only in terms of benefits, impersonally conceived, but also in relation to the patient's own sense of what he wants and whether he is able to choose. Nursing ethics, as we have noted, tends to start from the perspective of the patient (using the autonomy principle) in determining what treatment and care should be given to the patient. This tendency for one group of health care workers to use one model and another to select a different and sometimes opposing model augurs well for lively debate and exchange of ideas. Yet, because of the relative imbalance between the views and opinions of the medical beneficence model against the values of the nursing autonomous model, what could be a fruitful discussion of important matters of patient welfare can end up as frustrating, bad-tempered exchanges of prejudices and personal biases from either side.

Tension exists most obviously where there is doubt about the benefit of the usual treatment, where nursing staff feel that the patient's individual circumstances, values and beliefs have not been taken into consideration and where the expressed wishes of the patient are either being overruled or being ignored on the grounds of incompetence or limited autonomy. Yarling and McElmurry (1986) have identified a number of clinical situations where the conflict between the beneficence and autonomy models are most obvious. These include

care of patients in pain, cardiopulmonary resuscitation, withholding or withdrawing of life-sustaining treatment, . . . use of placebos, harmful care by another practitioner, and professional control of information.

(Yarling and McElmurry 1986, p. 64)

In order to understand something of the origin and nature of these problems we must first consider **paternalism** as it issues from the beneficence model and explore how considerations of **reduced autonomy** and **limited competence** influence the decision making process of doctors, nurses and patients.

4.7 PATERNALISM

Paternalism occurs where the explicit or implicit wishes of a person are overruled or disregarded in the choice of a course of action directed at the good of that person (cf. Beauchamp and Childress, 1983, pp. 170–171). Thus paternalism in deliberation involves giving greater weight to considerations supported by the principle of beneficence than to considerations backed by the principle of autonomy. Common examples of paternalistic acts are suicide interventions when patients are resistant, resuscitation of patients who have requested no further efforts, controlling information to patients either by withholding it or deceiving the patient by giving false information, engaging in various strategies of concealment in psychotherapy, forcible invasion of the body through surgery and telling small lies and engaging in deceptions which are intended to encourage the patient.

Komrad (1983) argues that paternalism is an inevitable characteristic of the doctor's relationship with the patient as all illness represents a state of diminished autonomy. Given this, limited forms of paternalism, aimed at restoring and maximizing the patient's autonomy are entirely acceptable. There is a duality in human nature: on the one hand, people are autonomous and responsible; on the other hand, they are in need of comfort, protection and support when their decision-making capacity is reduced by anxiety, worry or illness. This duality makes dilemmas inevitable. Given the patient's disadvantaged and vulnerable position in relation to the professional, one must ask whether and how the autonomous decision-making capacity of patients is to be preserved.

McNeil's (1981) study showed that what patients valued in relation to deciding courses of treatment for cancer of the larynx differed sharply from the values entering into medical deliberation. She found that patients' attitudes toward morbidity and survival were not their only consideration. Such attitudes can vary significantly from patient to patient, which seems to suggest that decisions based on the notion of 'clinical judgement' and the doctor's experience of similar cases as a guide to what is best for the particular case in hand is not acceptable. It is difficult to justify a professional's making a decision on behalf of a patient without close scrutiny of the individual patient's own values and their understanding of their own life story, of their illness, and of the significance of their illness for their life story.

Paternalism is easiest to defend in situations where the patient's autonomy is reduced and where the prospect of a good outcome (as defined by the professional) can be improved only by the health professional. Paternalism in cases of reduced autonomy is sometimes called **weak paternalism**. **Strong paternalism**, by contrast, occurs when the wishes of a patient, reckoned to be capable of making autonomous decisions, are overriden to prevent harm to the patient or to benefit them.

Weak paternalism is defended on the ground that, while patients may be able to make autonomous decisions regarding a range of self-care activities such as selection of food, choice of clothes to wear and so on, they are often unable to assimilate the information necessary to make major medical decisions regarding their future welfare. In such cases, it is argued, the professional is obliged to intervene and make the best possible decision on behalf of the patient in view of their compromised ability.

Paternalistic behaviour is thus characterized by the professional acting on behalf of and in the best interest of the patient. They are permitted to do this by the role conferred upon them as professionals, their authority based on the belief that they act always in the best interest of the patient, and their having the sensitivity and commitment to see the situation from the patient's point of view. However, we have noted that the beneficence model's stress on promoting value – the patient's welfare – may be at odds with the autonomy model's focus on the patient's autonomy. Tensions may develop, particularly in areas of judgements regarding the quality of life, the utility of certain treatments and the individual's conception of a dignified life or death.

Another tension relates to the fact that decision-making in medical care is invariably discussed in terms of doctors and their patient; third parties – other health care staff and relatives of the patient – are regarded as incidental to the proceedings. The distortion created by this view has repercussions in many areas of direct patient care, particularly where nursing staff do not agree with certain medical decisions, or where information is being withheld by one group but is desired by another. Again, the discrepancies between the beneficence model, as utilized by the medical profession, and the autonomy model, as advocated by the nursing profession, reinforces the problems created within certain clinical situations where what the patient wants (or might want) is not what they get.

4.8 REDUCED AUTONOMY AND LIMITED COMPETENCE

Nurses often defend their right to challenge medical decisions on the grounds that they are in a good position to judge the mental, emotional and physical capacity of their patients. They also claim to be able to get a better sense of the patient's values and conception of how to live because of the close intimate contact they have with them. Thus discussions of the nature of the patient's illness or disability, its consequences and how it might affect the patient's sense of himself arise quite naturally from the everyday encounters between the patient and the nurse. One can begin to see the handicapping effect of any unilateral medical decision that prohibits communication of the patient's health status when the nurse, by virtue of her intimate relationship with the patient, may indeed be the best judge of what he really should be told and how he should be supported through the experience.

A similar problem may arise when patients are classified as incapable of making autonomous decisions or as having limited competence. Again if the decision is based only on medical considerations, derived from a particular perspective without considering other observations, then the resulting treatments may not be acceptable to several members of the health care team, never mind the patient or their relatives.

Patients' levels of autonomy can be thought of as located on a continuum with independent decision-making autonomous patients at one end and dependent patients with no decisional capacities – for example, the profoundly mentally handicapped – at the other. The autonomy model is appropriate for patients at one end of the continuum whilst the beneficence model is appropriate for patients at the other end. The majority of patients have levels of autonomy somewhere between the two ends. Moreover, they will sometimes want to exercise their autonomy and sometimes be quite happy for someone else to make decisions for them. A possibility to explore, therefore, is that health professionals will usually be maintaining some blend of paternalism and non-paternalism. At any time the then-current blend will be at some point on a continuum whose end points are pure paternalism and pure nonpaternalism.

There is an obvious need for continuous feedback between the practitioners and the patient so that the balance between paternalism and nonpaternalism can be frequently updated and fine-tuned. This reflects the dynamic nature of the practitioner-patient relationship in terms of both its clinical and its moral progress. Szasz and Hollender (1956) first described the dynamics of this therapeutic relationship within the medical context. They described it as a 'process in that the patient may change not only in terms of his symptoms but also in the way in which he wishes to relate to his doctor'. They identify three models corresponding to different segments of the autonomy – dependence continuum:

Activity–passivity model

- where the patient is inert and the doctor does things without consent or dissent, for example unconscious patients, emergency cases, the profoundly handicapped.

Guidance–cooperation model

- where the doctor is active only as a guide and co-operator to the patient and where the patient exercises his choice for the most part, for example patients temporarily distracted by anxiety who need to be guided for a time until their decisions can be free of such distinctions.

Mutual–participation model

- where the doctor and patient are equal and mutually independent. Here the doctor helps the patient help himself.

Some nursing models reflect this dynamic relationship between the nurse and the patient. For example, Orem's (1980) wholly compensatory, partly compensatory and supportive–educative categories relate quite readily to Szasz and Hollender's (1956) model. The ethical decision-making role of the patient and nurse are more implied in this model, however, with the major focus being on the actions of the nurse.

Siegler (1977) has attempted to illustrate the close connection between the clinical factors determining medical decisions and a number of morally relevant factors that doctors assess when determining whether to respect the wishes of critically ill patients. In effect, he was attempting to locate them on the paternalism–nonpaternalism continuum in the light of a number of clinical and ethical factors. Siegler (1977) identified six factors that influence doctors' decisions, including the patient's ability to make rational choices about care, the consistency of the choice with the patient's own values, the age and level of maturity of the patient, the nature of the illness, the attitudes and values of the doctor responsible for the decision, their religious and moral background and attitude towards life and death, and the clinical setting (whether a uni- or multidisciplinary perspective was being taken).

Underpinning these factors was the requirement for the practitioner to establish a sense of the baseline personality of the individual. This provides a standard against which the practitioner can compare the current behaviour and decisions of the patient to their past values and preferences.

Siegler sees this expression of the patient's stable values as a critical factor in determining their level of autonomy and in assuring a level of coherence between current behaviour and actions, past events, and future expectations. The challenge, as he sees it, is more than permitting patients to choose; rather it is facilitating the person in making decision that represent them most faithfully by expressing settled preferences and beliefs as contrasted with actions and choices motivated by anxieties, fears or desires.

This orientation to the patient's own values, self-understanding and conception of how to live, together with a respect for their personal biography, is perhaps more consistently articulated in nursing models and theories. Whilst the doctor–patient relationship may have respect for persons as a fundamental tenet guiding medical practice, we have already sensed the insidiousness of the beneficence model which can all too readily replace what the patient says he wants with what he ought to have and what is best for him. Indeed, a patient can suffer a reduction in autonomy by the very fact that the values and beliefs that he adheres to are not those gaining precedence in the beneficence model.

A person's autonomy may be diminished by such factors as inadequate knowledge, lack of understanding, internal constraints (such as pain, fear or depression), or external ones (such as pressure from relative, the effects of the illness, prognosis, treatment, or hospitalization – cf. Beauchamp and McCullough, 1984, p. 116). Obviously there are few decisions made that are free of all of these factors. Practitioners must be able to recognize and take account of the impact any one of these items may be having on the patient. If overruling a patient's wishes is to be justified at all then the claim that the patient's autonomy is diminished has to be supported by reference to some such factor. But it is plainly unsatisfactory if such judgements can be made by one member of the health care team on behalf of others and without consultation with the patient and exploration of the patient's expectations. And it would be a mistake to suppose that paternalism on the grounds of diminished autonomy is justified by the mere presence of one of the listed factors. For example, a person may succeed in reaching an autonomous decision even if there *is* family pressure on them.

Care may be needed also to avoid the natural mistake of inferring general reduced autonomy from localized diminution of competence. With such groups as the hospitalized elderly, the disabled, and the mentally ill, diminution in certain skills may prompt the assumption of inability to make decisions regarding other parts of their life. Beauchamp and McCullough (1984, p. 126) note that compromised states do not justify the person's subjection to whatever form of medical benefit another might think good for him. They cite the example of a case involving a committed mental patient whose right to refuse treatment (in this case the forced injection of psychotropic medication) was upheld by the courts. The medical argument was that if the patient had to be committed to the hospital against his will then there was sufficient justification to treat the patient against his will. The courts however took a different view and argued that incompetence in one area in life did not necessarily mean that the person was incapable of making any autonomous decisions. Such decisions may in fact help preserve what little dignity remains to them in stark institutional settings. If limited competence is to be a reason for paternalistic action, the deficiency has to be a deficiency in the relevant kind of competence.

Meisel and Roth (1981) have identified a number of factors to help determine a person's level of competence to make autonomous decisions. These concern decision, reasons, understanding, and conclusions. They include the abilities to evidence preferences and communicate decisions, to give reasons for a particular choice, to give reasons which are rational, and to take account of a reasonable weighting of risks and benefits, to understand alternatives and understand information provided by the professionals, and to arrive at a choice that a reasonable person would have arrived at. This last factor is questionable. It means in effect that if the patient were to choose what a reasonable person would not choose in similar circumstances then the patient lacks the relevant competence. Thus a judgement about competence is based on the outcome of the patient's deliberation rather than the process by which it was reached. This makes it too easy to discount a value judgement merely on the strength of its differing from one's own or from most other people's. It therefore seems better to require that bizarre choices be placed on an equal footing with other choices unless some defect in the process by which they were reached can be specified.

The question who is in charge requires consideration of individual autonomy and professional obligations to do no harm and to provide positive benefits. It also requires consideration of what happens when people become patients and how their increased vulnerability affects their ability to make rational decisions or even retain certain skills and competencies that they exercised quite regularly in their everyday lives. Again, the potential conflict between the medical profession and its view of the world (shaped primarily by the beneficence model), the nursing profession's perspective (shaped by the autonomy model), and somewhere in the middle the patient and his family trying valiantly to make some sort of sense of the world that illness or disability has propelled them into is a poignant reminder of the reality that such complex situations need careful consideration and open discussion before each party can be convinced of the wisdom of their decision.

No matter what part of the paternalism–nonpaternalism continuum one finds oneself on, an essential requirement already identified by Siegler

(1977), Szasz and Hollender (1956), and Orem (1980) is the need to have a clear picture of what the patient really values about his life and how he makes sense of the things happening to him. Pellegrino (1979) calls it the patient's value history where decisions regarding the diagnosis and treatment could be made consistent with the value history. Veatch (1981, pp. 209–210) refers to the moral history of the individual which must include a determination of the patient's values (judgements of good and harm) in relation to the beneficence model and how these are weighed. The role of the family members in piecing together the patient's moral history is also seen as central and the practitioner's job is to collate this information in order to help in the decision-making process.

4.9 THE CASE STUDY REVISITED

Let us now reconsider the student nurse's dilemma concerning whether she should encourage Mr D to have his pacemaker replaced when he has stated that he could see no reason for prolonging his life by undergoing such a procedure. The student nurse had made a preliminary judgement that she would set this as one of her nursing goals but she was infringing the patient's right to choose. How could she satisfy herself that she was doing the right thing and indeed what was the right thing to do?

Obviously there are a number of underlying ethical principles that she has to consider. We have already discussed the dilemma in terms of the conflict between the patient's right to decide (autonomy model) and the nurse's sense of obligation to bring about the best outcome for the patient (beneficence model). What we need is more information about whether Mr D is a fully autonomous individual or whether his lack of desire to live following his wife's death is really a manifestation of depression and grieving which is influencing his ability to make a rational decision about his own welfare. Does the student nurse know enough about Mr D's own value and belief system to construct a moral history of him which would help her understand why he does not seem to want to preserve his own life? Does she know whether his decision is based on sufficient accurate information regarding the risks and benefits of the treatment and can she be assured that the outcome of his decision is well balanced and rational?

The patient's moral history

The student nurse's piecing together of Mr D's moral history occurred in several stages over her period of contact with him. His present situation reflects a history of loss and altered self-image, his wife dead, his existence confined to a nursing home and his health status slowly deteriorating. However, she has had an opportunity to observe how he chooses to organize his activities of daily living and notes that he values his independence and his ability to go for his walk each afternoon. His Jewish heritage also means that he places high value on life and one's responsibility to live it to the full. The student reported that Mr D's conversation, in discussion of these issues, indicated that he had a distorted perception of what was involved in replacing a pacemaker. This led her to consider Mr D's level of competence and whether he was capable of making autonomous decisions.

The patient's level of autonomy and competence

The discovery that Mr D's decision not to have his pacemaker replaced was based on false information led the student to consider whether the problem lay with Mr D's inability to understand the accurate information given to him or whether he had been given inaccurate information. The records showed that the medical and nursing staff had repeatedly attempted to persuade him to have the pacemaker replaced. Was his distorted perception due to some internal constraint such as depression or did it have an external source, perhaps related to the unhappiness he experienced in having to live by himself in the nursing home? Was Mr D sufficiently competent to make a decision about his own welfare? The evidence before her led the student to consider the possibility that Mr D was unable to weigh the potential risks and benefits of the treatment and thus reach a considered conclusion. He was demonstrating a general inability to understand the nature of the situation and as such was not making the most sensible decision about his welfare.

From this the student concluded that she would have to go through the risks and benefits involved in the procedure and at the same time incorporate the now explicit values and beliefs the patient had regarding what he wanted to happen to him.

The student nurse's values and decision-making process

The student was forced back to consider her own values and conception of how to live early on in the encounter when her notion of what was best for Mr D was at odds with his own. Elements of the beneficence model had become part of her thinking – preservation of life was a most important goal, intervention and making decisions on behalf of the patient were justified sometimes and, above all, the practitioner should do no harm. She tried to get a measure of these considerations by weighing up the risks and benefits involved in the case. She reckoned that Mr D had three options: (a) he could continue to do nothing about the pacemaker, (b) he could wait until he got into serious cardiac difficulties and then have the pacemaker replaced, (c) he could have the pacemaker replaced before his cardiac status worsened. If he chose not to have the pacemaker replaced the consequences of his actions would be either: maintenance of current cardiac status and functional capacity, a gradual decline in cardiac status and functional capacity or precipitation of serious cardiac dysfunction and severe limitation of activity.

Given the prior discussions that had taken place the student was able to accept that the replacement of the pacemaker from a risk-benefit analysis perspective was the most sensible thing to do. But how was she going to get the patient to see it and what if he continued to refuse to be persuaded? Would she then be ready to accept that the professional staff's position was more acceptable than the patient's and that he should have the treatment regardless of his wishes? This was the most difficult situation to resolve as the whole notion of respecting the patient and acknowledging his right to determine what would happen to him was central to her understanding of the nurse–patient relationship.

Aspects of the nurse–patient relationship

The resolution of the student's dilemma occurred as she was able to unravel the different parts of the situation within the context of her relationship with Mr D. Early on she had faced the issue of who actually owned the problem. She had tended to set her nursing objective in terms of getting the patient to agree to change his pacemaker. She then came to realize that the issue was not so much one of coercing the patient to do it but more of helping Mr D to examine his own values and assisting him to make an informed decision. This growing awareness of the negotiating involved in the decision-making process led to a much closer relationship between the nurse and Mr D. The nurse's role was one of facilitation of the patient's ability to explore his values and check his understanding of the situation. It was also necessary for the nurse first to communicate an empathic understanding of Mr D's perception of his situation before offering him suggestions for seeing it differently.

In Mr D's case this turned out to yield an outcome that both were content with. Ryden (1978, p. 706) concludes:

> Although the student's goal had changed from that of convincing Mr D to replace the pacemaker to that of assisting him to make an informed decision about it, she was delighted to report to the group that Mr D had decided to have the pacemaker replaced and was scheduled for surgery in the near future.

4.10 DISCUSSION

The resolution of the problem in this way illustrates the importance of the personal relationship between the nurse and the patient. It reflects aspects of the caring relationship described in Chapter Three where the nurse's willingness to get to know the patient was an important component in building up trust and empathy. However, it is important to remember that within the dynamics of this relationship there would also be a number of roles and responsibilities of other professionals and third party interests. Considering the nurse–patient relationship in abstraction helps us to identify a number of key factors that will influence the decision-making process for both parties involved. But we cannot be confident that the process will be unaffected if there are different pressures coming to bear on either the patient or the nurse.

Take the situation where Mr D and the student are two actors within a larger scenario where the consultant has determined what is best, where Mr D's relatives are in agreement with the medical decision, and where the nursing staff generally conform to the wishes of the doctor. Then the student nurse's concern over whether Mr D should be allowed to choose is a rather academic question. Her sense of powerlessness would be matched only by that of Mr D; both of them would have to either accept the inevitability of the decision or fight against it. The dominant values in the system reinforce the professional hierarchy where doctors are commonly taken to know what is best for the patient and where the observations, sensitivities and perceptions of other professionals are subordinated.

Fradd (1988) provides a forceful example of the importance of those observations, sensitivities and perceptions. She tells the story of Gavin, a three-year-old who from the age of ten months had been suffering from haemolytic uraemic syndrome. He required frequent hospital visits and quite complicated medical and nursing interventions to control his illness. Following one particularly bad episode it became clear to the medical team that the way forward was to plan for a kidney transplant.

After careful consideration and against the advice of the paediatrician, both parents, supported by the extended family, decided not to proceed. They asked that all active treatment should be stopped and they also requested that the nurse most directly involved in the case (the author of the article) should convey their reasons to the consultant and nursing staff if they (the parents) either were unable to do so or were not present when discussions took place. They identified the strain of seeing their son suffer and the constant pressure of being both nurse and parent as factors which outweighed the slim chance of a resolution of Gavin's illness. Yet the vulnerability and anguish they felt regarding their decision were acute and they needed help to enable them to view the situation from the multiple perspectives of parents, guardians, carers, disappointed and worn out individuals and people in need of comfort themselves. This was possible only within an open and trusting relationship where the parents felt under-stood and able to articulate the fears and concerns they were having.

The active involvement of patients in their own care, and of parents in the care of their sick children, is one approach that has been used to help people feel in control of what is happening to them or their dependants. The psychological and emotional struggle of carers having to face and accept the death of their loved ones is an extremely complex situation to deal with. The nurse, often in closest contact with both patient and carers, is party to the struggle that often goes on. She has to decide how this information is interpreted and fed back to other members of the health care team and indeed presented to the patient and carers themselves for affirmation and clarification.

The value attributed to this sort of information and whether it is con-sidered when weighing up the goods and harms of a particular intervention is a debate we will enter into more fully in Chapter Five. We have noted some of the issues that might lead some individuals to select a particular intervention while others would support a more laissez-faire approach. We have seen the heightened dilemmas that emerge when choices made run counter to the autonomous wishes of the patient.

We cannot solve the dilemmas simply by saying that we should always do what the patient wishes. Even strong advocates of patient autonomy will find themselves exercising power over patients in the most subtle of ways (consider the effect of ward routines, visiting restrictions, and a whole range of unobtrusive processes that essentially neutralize the indi-vidual in exercising choice). We can perhaps avoid being seduced into exploiting the inequality of the practitioner–patient relationship by the constant reminder that patients are unique individuals with their own moral histories (Veatch, 1981, p. 209) with whom we have the privilege to engage at a particularly difficult time in their life story. Such a percep-tion may help us kindle respect for them as people so that we engage with them as people rather than objects. This is our professional obligation and one of the few checks that we can use to evaluate whether we are capable of making a judgement – a cautious, tentative, and corrigible judgement – about what is best for another person.

FIVE

Interprofessional relationships – nurses and doctors

5.1 INTRODUCTION

An experienced nurse, working in the outpatients department of her local hospital, recently recounted two situations where she felt she had been badly treated by her medical colleague. In one case, the consultant shouted at the nurse because she could not provide him with an extra nurse to collect the patient's details and another to act as chaperone. What the nurse objected most strongly to was that the consultant shouted at her in front of the patient.

In the second case, the nurse was asked to 'get rid' of patients waiting to see the consultant as he was running behind schedule with his clinic and had a pressing appointment elsewhere. Here the doctor was asking the nurse, in effect, to deceive the patients in some way that would permit him to keep his appointment and which would maintain his good reputation in the eyes of his patients.

Do these cases illustrate the nature of the unequal relationship between doctors and nurses? If not, then they are simply two isolated cases, the situation is not a common one, and it could equally have been the other way round (with the nurse scolding the doctor in front of patients and the nurse telling the doctor to get rid of waiting patients). Among equals, such behaviour would be unusual and rather shocking. Readers who do find these incidents extraordinary will not share this chapter's working assumption that there are at present serious inequalities in the relationship between doctors and nurses. If some readers are unsurprised by the anecdotes, this shows that these readers take considerable inequality for granted. Only considerable domination would permit rudeness and require one person to compromise their moral views (by deceiving the patient) in order to protect the other person.

Is this state of affairs something we should be concerned about? Does it indeed matter if some doctors are rude in front of patients and will it really make any difference if the nurse has to cover up for her colleagues now and again? Whilst we can analyse this situation in a satisfactory way at the level of interpersonal relationship and individual character traits there are also important ethical issues, concerning shared background assumptions and expectations, that have wider implications. We need to explore the nature of relationships between health care professionals (and particularly between doctors and nurses) because caring requires not only an openness and receptiveness to the patient's needs but also a readiness to reflect on the way the professionals make judgements about what is best for the patient.

Thus, instead of starting from a consideration of what nurses and doctors dislike about each other, or even admire and respect in each other's practice, we attempt to explore the nature of the doctor–nurse relationship within the context of trying to find out what is best for the patient. Our exploration takes the form of a case study. A clinical example from an acute paediatric surgical ward is set out in section 5.4 below and used to illustrate some of the underlying moral issues and principles involved in a common patient care situation. But before proceeding to the case we need to remind ourselves of some of the factors that affect doctors' and nurses' perceptions of their own roles.

In an analysis of medical and nursing codes of professional conduct Campbell (1984a, p. 6) identifies the common guiding principle as the concept of service to mankind. In the World Medical Association's Declaration of Geneva (reprinted in Beauchamp and Childress, 1983, pp. 330–331) the doctor solemnly pledges to consecrate his life to the service of humanity. Nurses too, following the International Code of Nursing Ethics which was formally adopted by the International Council for Nurses in 1953 (later versions are reprinted in Campbell, 1984a; Beauchamp and Childress 1983, and elsewhere), have identified service to mankind as their primary function and the reason for the existence of the nursing profession.

In such broad principles as service to mankind and respect for human life there is little disagreement between professional groups. But when we begin to consider how such universal principles are applied within the context of professional norms and values we find interesting divergences.

5.2 MEDICINE – PROFESSIONAL AND ORGANIZATIONAL VALUES

The moral obligation of the doctor has been summarized by the beneficence model of patient care. In the Hippocratic tradition, individuals choosing to enter the profession of medicine were committed men, set apart from and above other members of society, charged with a moral purpose to use their specialized skills and knowledge for the benefit of their patients. And above all they were to keep from doing any harm to those in their care.

The beneficence model for the most part fits comfortably into the traditions of medical thought, whereby an understanding of the patient's best interests could be gained exclusively from the perspective of medicine. Beauchamp and McCullough (1984, p. 22) describe it thus:

> The practice of medicine issues from the repository of tested knowledge, skills and experience constituting the science and art of care, the alleviation and prevention of disease and injury. So understood, it provides . . . an objective perspective on the patient's best interests. The goals of the medical enterprise, as well as duties and virtues of physicians, are expressed in terms of both goods that should be sought on behalf of patients and harms to be avoided.

In this respect the beneficence model, whilst pointing to obligations to provide necessary care to vulnerable patients, also supports the notion that the doctor is often in the best position to know what is the most appropriate care for the patient. Thus, acting in a paternalistic way towards patients (making decisions about treatment on their behalf, going against their expressed wishes if they are not compatible with the medical care view of what is best and choosing how much information to divulge) is a consequence of the beneficence model. By virtue of his moral obligation to his patients, the doctor has the privilege (sometimes) of overriding the wishes of his patient because he knows what is best.

As well as the special obligation and the knowledge just noted, the doctor must also have authority. If he knows what is best for his patient and society has entrusted him with the responsibility to do his best and above all do no harm to those in his care then he must be obeyed. The patient must obey him, those working for him must obey him, and he has the right to challenge any of their actions.

Such professional authority, based as it is on the knowledge and the moral responsibility of the doctor to provide the best care, is a very powerful force. This is manifested in the doctor's privilege to admit and discharge patients from hospitals (see Brewer, 1988), ratify the classification of some people as ill and of others as hypochondriacs, and initiate treatments that have life-threatening consequences.

The organization of medical work conforms to this autonomous image: doctors, for the most part, are independent professionals, regulating their own standards and practice, using professional colleagues as judges of each other's practice and the doctor's right to confidentiality in analysing cases.

Within this ostensibly egalitarian framework, a rigid hierarchical structure operates. Bosk (1979) has described it in relation to how surgeons deal with surgical errors – both their own and their subordinates'. In a fascinating study of the social organization of medical practice he found that surgeons classified errors into four categories – technical, judgemental, normative and quasi-normative errors. Technical and judgemental errors related to the experience, skill, and knowledge of the doctor, and these were seen as inevitable consequences of an apprentice's training. If they occurred in experienced practitioners they were seen as faults that can be ridiculed. More serious for all concerned were the normative errors where the surgeon had failed to discharge his role obligations conscientiously. If the surgeon had been lazy or had not diligently carried out his work then this was taken to be a sign that he did not have the moral fibre to make a good surgeon (Bosk, 1979, p. 51). Quasi-normative errors were less serious; they were mistakes made by new staff and consisted in not following the eccentricities of the particular consultant. Doctors who continued to make such errors were seen as deliberately obstructive and thus were seen as having made mistakes as serious as normative errors.

Thus within the ostensibly collegial system of medical practice a rigid hierarchy exists where more experienced practitioners exert authority and influence over their less experienced colleagues. Such power and authority also extends to medical specialties with the stereotyped pecking order of high-technology, life-and-death medicine attracting most prestige and adulation and the low-technology, chronic care specialties such as care of the elderly, general practice and so on being less prestigious.

In these latter areas, where the contrast between the medical role of caring and curing has been less stark, there has been a growing emergence of a more patient-focused approach to medical practice. As noted in section 4.3, this approach, called the patient-autonomy model, alters the way professionals think about patients, about situations involving patients and about the relationships between patients and health care workers. It involves a collection of shared assumptions, dispositions, and expectations. It has at its base such ethical principles as respect for persons, never using someone merely as a means to an end, and the recognition and valuing of a range of participants in the decision-making process.

By embracing the values of the patient-autonomy model – or at least moving some way towards recognizing how it affects practice – the medical profession is faced with two major organizational issues. One is the question of how they (continue to) facilitate the patient in making the best decision they can about their care. The second – and perhaps more contentious – issue is how doctors negotiate their working relationship with other health care workers – and in this instance particularly with nurses – to promote the principles of mutual respect, to resist using others only as means to an end, and to involve all relevant people in the decision-making process.

5.3 NURSING – PROFESSIONAL AND ORGANIZATIONAL VALUES

The presence of the medical beneficence model and, more recently, the emerging patient autonomy model has had a marked influence on the way the nursing profession has described its practice. Like its medical counterpart, the nursing profession had found itself increasingly having to accommodate two starkly opposing value systems. These can be identified by their predominant characteristics as the traditional obedience model and – within the nursing literature – the patient autonomy model. What is interesting to note at this point is how within the context of the parallel medical models, the obedience model fits snugly into the medical beneficence model perpetuating the hierarchical, dominance-submission approach while both the medical and nursing perspectives on the patient autonomy model should embrace the same values, namely those articulated above.

It is not difficult to see the advantage of promoting such virtues as 'unquestioning obedience' (Dock, 1917: Pearce, 1969) and loyalty to the doctor or as Moore (1935) more elegantly puts it as being 'a faithful servant to a master' – when the predominant ideology within health care was traditionally that of medical beneficence. The nurse, in this context, was rightly seen as the physician's assistant, diligent, hardworking, trustworthy and loyal. She was conscientious in her duties and used her special nurturing skills to provide comfort to patients so that the real work of medicine might not be impeded.

Early nursing codes reinforce this subservient role. As recently as 1965, the International Council of Nurses' Code for Nurses stated that 'The nurse is under an obligation to carry out the physician's orders intelligently and loyally . . .' (This statement was later revised in the 1973 version to read 'the nurse sustains a cooperative relationship with the co-workers . . .'). Traces can also be seen in debates on whether nurses, either as individuals or professionals, have any right to refuse to participate in unethical procedures. Curtin and Flaherty (1982, p. 83) illustrate this point, quoting from Gustafson (1973):

In an article discussing the deliberate starvation of an infant born with Down's Syndrome and duodenal atresia, the author stated that the nurses' duties were '. . . to carry out the order of the physician. Even if they conscientiously believed that the orders they were executing were immoral, they could not radically reverse the order of events; they could not perform surgery. It was their lot to be the immediate participants in a sad event but to be powerless to alter its course. *They are the instruments of the physicians.* They have no right of conscientious objection, at least not in this set of circumstances.' (The emphasis is Curtin's.)

A striking feature of the quoted passage is the apparent inference from the subordinate knowledge and skill of the nurse ('could not perform surgery') to a subordinate moral role in relation to the doctor ('instruments of the physicians', 'no right of conscientious objection'). This might be tolerable if, as Gustafson (1973) seems to suggest, the role of the nurse is that of medical assistant: it is less likely that assistants will object to the judgements of their superiors. The medical assistant role, however, does not rest easily in the hearts and minds of nurses. For nurses to be medical assistants is always to be assistants, not apprentices where some day they too can exercise choice and control. But what is more distressing is that in this role nurses, as Yarling and McElmurry (1986) have argued, are not free to be moral because they are deprived of the free exercise of moral agency.

Yarling and McElmurry (1986) reinforce the argument put forward by Davis and Aroskar (1978, pp. 42–43) who identified several organizational and social constraints in hospitals that impede the ethical practice of nurses. These include 'the role and social position of the physician and the nurse in the hospital's social system . . . the role and power of the nursing leadership in the system, sexism and paternalism'. Several case studies illustrating aspects of the above factors are included in Yarling and McElmurry's 1986 paper (pp. 68–69). Many of the examples concern conflicts over the nurse's right to practice nursing and make independent judgements regarding the patient's welfare. The infringement of the nurse's right to practice nursing can come from several sources – notably the hospital organizational decisions and medical decisions that run counter to what the nurse sees to be what is best for the patient.

Once the notion that nurses practice nursing (rather than medicine or a watered down version of it) is made explicit, the need for a new way of looking at the complementary roles of nurses, doctors, and patients becomes apparent. The gradual change in emphasis in the ANA nursing code over a 25-year span from obeying doctors' orders to taking responsibility for one's own actions illustrates the change. Most other professional nursing organizations have declared in equally direct ways the emerging autonomous role of the nurse and her professional right to practice nursing in the manner best suited to the needs of her patients (see for example, Canadian Nurses Association (1980) and Royal College of Nursing Guidelines (1986)).

Such declarations or professional independence must be justified on grounds other than self-aggrandizement or professional imperialism on the part of nurses. Curtin and Flaherty (1982, p. 87) have summarized the appropriate grounds succinctly in terms of the nature of the nurse–patient relationship and what it does to the patient. They argue that disease or disability of any kind magnifies the human needs any individual will have; it also creates new needs and can render the individual vulnerable on a number of fronts. It reduces human autonomy, reducing the individual's ability to express himself and act as he wishes; it alters the individual's ability to make choices and consequently can augment the power of others over that person's needs, desires and wishes.

Such observations have led nurses to commit themselves to serving patients in a special way through the practice of nursing. Curtin has identified four promises implicitly made by nurses:

> Nurses have promised to help those who are ill to regain their health, those who are healthy to maintain their health, those who cannot be cured to maximize their potential and those who are dying to live as fully as possible until their deaths.
>
> (Curtin and Flaherty, 1982, p. 98)

These promises overlap with four principles – of promoting health, preventing illness, restoring health and alleviating suffering – identified by the International Council of Nurses (1986). The nurse also promises to carry personal responsibility for nursing practice and for maintaining competence by continual learning. She is exhorted to maintain the highest professional standards, use her own judgement as to her level of professional competence in accepting responsibility for patient care and should cooperate with co-workers (ICN, 1973). The UKCC *Code of Professional Conduct* (1984) similarly reflects these sentiments.

In some respects such exhortations may remind us of the ancient Hippocratic Oath and the various World Medical Association declarations of modern times (see Gillon, 1986 pp. 9–13). We may wonder whether nursing is choosing to parody medical practice in its promises and professional codes. Yet it is important to remember the sharp contrasts that often exist between nursing and medical dilemmas. Nurses very often find themselves defending the patient's right to refuse treatment or to be told the truth about their condition. This can be construed as nurses being disobedient to medical orders. But it can also be seen as the proposal of a view – equally legitimate and equally deserving of consideration – as to what is best for the patient. Instead of viewing things in terms of the beneficence-paternalistic model, the nurse is more comfortable with the perspective of the patient autonomy model.

We have already identified many reasons for this variation in viewpoints. The nurse, in performing nursing, engages more closely with the individual, acts as a support and companion (Campbell, 1984a, p. 49) to the patient, and all the time seeks to restore them to a level of experiencing the world which is acceptable and tolerable to them. For nurses there is little talk about cure; it is more about restoration. The nurse–patient relationship is therefore more naturally based on partnership and continuing negotiation. The patient has to trust the nurse in order to be supported through a number of experiences; but the support the nurse provides is safeguarded from becoming overpowering and autocratic by her allegiance to the principle of patient autonomy.

The exercise of a patient's right to choose is seen at every level of the nurse–patient encounter, from negotiating routines related to activities of daily living to making decisions about their treatment or lack of it. However, the honouring of that right is not guaranteed by working arrangements. The nurse continues to have the option of setting aside her obligation to the patient at any moment and choosing to comply with organizational rules or requests (orders) from other professional groups which will compromise, even if only in a very small way, the rights of the patient. If she takes this option then she begins to undermine her relationship with the patient; in the extreme case she may find that, having done something against her professional and personal conscience, she is unable to continue caring for the patient. Thus the change from an obedience model to a patient autonomy model is at best imperfect. Such a change is complete only when, as well as the individual's practice being shaped by the assumptions and dispositions characteristic of the new model, each individual expects the others' practice to be so shaped, so that the influence of the model on practice is continually confirmed and consolidated.

The effective transition from the traditional obedience model of nursing to a new patient autonomy model is fraught with problems, not least because the traditional model complemented the beneficence model so beautifully. The tension within the practice of medicine itself between doing what is best for the patient (beneficence model) and recognizing their right to choose (patient autonomy model) illustrates in a small way the more obvious problems that will ensue if one professional group, with a tradition of obedience and subservience, then appears to be advocating an approach to medical care which favours the patient autonomy model. It will often be seen as simply preposterous. The crux of the matter is that one group of professionals cannot change the focus and orientation of the way they provide care without obtaining the consent and co-operation of their colleagues. Unfortunately, change in the nursing camp is too often construed as 'nurses-wanting-to-play-doctor' with patient-centred motives merely providing the vehicle for attack. Similarly, any medical approach to involve patients and other professionals in more active decision-making is viewed with scepticism – a scepticism which the sceptic often sees as justified when the genuine offer of a more democratic approach to care is met with suspicion, vacillation, indecision, and an unwillingness to take on the extra responsibility.

It is all too easy, for the sake of contrast, to portray doctors as male-chauvinistic, arrogant, unfeeling and paternalistic and nurses as subservient, ineffectual and for the most part incapable of taking on the weighty responsibility of patient care. But knowing what is best for a patient is not about making one major decision; rather the reality of caring for people requires many repeated and reassessed decisions, constant evaluation of the situation, consideration of multiple perspectives, careful analysis of the facts and insightful dissection of the fiction that makes up a patient's story.

5.4 A CASE FOR STUDY

Nine year old Brian had been diagnosed at birth as having a mild case of spina bifida. Although generally in good health, he had never been able to gain control of his bladder and this meant frequent trips to and from the local children's hospital. Brian's last hospitalization had been for the insertion of a Dacron implant in the neck of his bladder. His parents had been told that a procedure of this sort, whereby the tightening of the bladder neck allows the patient to begin to gain control over his voiding pattern, was quite normal for boys like Brian. It would be better to have this operation before puberty, Brian's parents were told, so that he could get used to intermittently catheterizing himself. It was also better for him in that he would no longer have to wear incontinence pads, he would not be prone to so many urinary tract infections and generally his quality of life would improve.

Brian, however, was rather unimpressed with the whole business. Despite his pleasant personality, the nurses noted the he was often withdrawn on the ward and sometimes noticed him acting quite aggressively towards the other, younger children. His mother was keen to get him out of pads and using a catheter, but, when asked about it, Brian told the nurses that he had not really minded wearing pads. When it came to teaching him to catheterize himself, Brian reluctantly went along with the nursing instructions. He was discharged two weeks after his operation.

A short time later, Brian was readmitted to the ward. His catheter had become blocked and he was passing stones. He was very frightened and was crying. The doctors saw him and confirmed that there were no major complications but recommended that he remain in hospital for a few days for observation. The ward sister, however, began to consider what had happened since Brian had gone home. She sensed by observing Brian's behaviour, particularly when he was with his mother, that his reluctance had something to do with a number of factors in the background. She therefore decided to call one of the clinical nurse specialists in the hospital to ask her advice. (The term 'clinical nurse specialist' was a relatively new one at the time, describing the roles of a small team of nurses within the paediatric hospital who specialized in caring for children with a range of complicated, long-term health problems.)

Sister Wells, whose background was in child psychiatry and paediatrics, had specialized in the care and management of children with bowel and bladder problems and was used peripatetically by the nursing staff in both the hospital and the neighbouring clinics and health centres. The ward sister, Sister Jones, discussed Brian's case with the clinical nurse specialist, Sister Wells. Sister Jones told Sister Wells that she did not have the time to try and get Brian to accept the intermittent catheterization regime. She acknowledged the difficulty of the case, which was due not only to Brian's last – painful – readmission but also to a number of underlying problems which she had detected in the relationship between mother and son. She said that it would be a pity if Brian had to go home with an indwelling catheter – the last resort as far as she was concerned – and that she would like Sister Wells to spend some time with Brian and his family both in the hospital and, more importantly, at home. Sister Wells agreed to have a chat with Brian and his mother and reported her observations in the nursing care plan.

Shortly after this conversation between ward sister and clinical nurse specialist, the doctor in charge of Brian's treatment (Mr White) examined him and decided that Brian had come as far as he could in hospital and therefore could be discharged that afternoon. At that point the ward sister said that in her opinion Brian was still not ready to go home, since they were not certain that he would continue to catheterize himself after discharge. She then mentioned her conversation with the clinical nurse specialist, saying that she had asked her to get involved in the case.

Mr White said that Sister Jones had no business asking for advice from someone without his permission, as Brian was his patient; Brian was his responsibility and he would not permit this clinical nurse specialist – whatever that was – to interfere with his patient. Sister Jones, by this time, was becoming quite animated and declared that if he had not discharged Brian so quickly the first time and had listened to them about the management problems they had anticipated then maybe there would have been no need for Brian to be readmitted. At this point Mr White, refusing to listen any more, reminded Sister Jones that he was in charge and said that Brian would be discharged that afternoon as clinically there was nothing more that could be done for him. Mr White then walked out of the ward.

Brian was discharged that afternoon.

When the incident was discussed with the nurses involved a number of issues emerged:

1 The nurses were generally unhappy with the care that Brian had received. They felt unfulfilled in the professional care they had provided and they found themselves being critical of their medical colleague for effectively discharging Brian before he ought (in the nurses' opinion) to have gone home.
2 They resented the fact that the surgeon had the power to overrule the nursing care that had been planned for Brian and they felt frustrated that Mr White and his colleagues would not listen to their ideas and refused to consider using the clinical nurse specialist.
3 They could not see a justification for Mr White's behaviour even, as they said, in terms of his aim of acting in the best interests of his patient. Even though the surgical procedure had been a success the original objective (namely Brian's being able to catheterize himself intermittently) had not been achieved.

5.5 MORAL ASPECTS OF THE CASE

This particular case reflects a range of problems inherent in the nurse–doctor relationship as it exists at present. The first issue to be raised is related to the autonomous positions of any professional group relative to the actions of other personnel and the welfare of the patient. Medical autonomy has its roots in the exercise of medical skills and knowledge of the good of the patient. Part of this condition requires the balancing of the doctor's judgement of what is best for the patient with the person's own value and belief system, and his exercise of his right to self determination. The doctor's moral obligation to do his best for his patient, and his obligation to work to promote the best interests of all his patients are most effectively executed when the practitioner displays personal qualities which reflect honesty and patience rather than self-advancement or conceit.

The idea of nursing autonomy has been gaining currency more recently because of the growing recognition that nurses practice nursing and that, in the execution of this function, they have a number of obligations to society and to individuals. Nurses exercise their function by engaging with members of society in order to meet various needs: protection from illness, promotion of health, alleviation of suffering, and restoration of health. Nursing skills and knowledge are used for restorative and supportive purposes, the nurse often being a vital help and companion to the patient. The relationship between the nurse and patient is based on partnership and negotiation where the wishes and request of the patient are the first lines of departure for the nurse to determine the best and most productive course of action. Sensitivity, compassion, fortitude and patience are the preferred character traits of people who choose to become nurses.

Both doctors and nurses seek to do their best for their patients; both seek to exercise their skills and knowledge in the best possible way, both are diligent and conscientious and both exercise a number of personal qualities in achieving such ends. Doctors are critical of nurses who do not carry out their orders, nurses accuse doctors of not considering the patient's point of view sufficiently when they make decisions; doctors believe that they are ultimately responsible for medical care (by which they mean total patient care); nurses seek recognition for their nursing contribution to total patient care and question the assertion that a medical decision is equivalent to a decision about the patient's total welfare.

Let us see how factors such as these enter into the moral arguments relating to the case of Brian. There are four possible hypotheses that we need to examine:

1. that both Mr White the surgeon and Sister Jones the ward sister were correct in their actions;
2. that Mr White was right and the nurses were wrong in what they were trying to do;
3. that Mr White was acting wrongly and Sister Jones correctly;
4. that there were wrongs on both sides, both Mr White and Sister Jones having dealt with the situation inappropriately.

We consider each of these in turn.

5.6 FIRST HYPOTHESES: DOCTORS RIGHT – NURSES RIGHT

Let us consider the case with reference to the hypothesis that both the medical and the nursing staff were justified in their actions. The supposition here is that the actions of both were morally unobjectionable.

This is probably the most difficult of our four hypotheses to sustain. We know that the overall desired outcome of care for Brian was that he should become independent in his elimination habits. Furthermore, longer term goals were that, before reaching the awkward stage of puberty, he reduce any potential problems in terms of socializing with his contemporaries and reduce any risks of urinary tract and kidney infections. The description of the case makes clear that this primary goal was not achieved on discharge and that no provision was made, particularly by the medical staff, to ensure that it be achieved. We are thus faced with the thought that even though the surgical intervention itself had been successful – there had been no complications – the follow-up treatment was deficient.

Nevertheless, the hypotheses fits well with some aspects of the case. The surgeon successfully carried out his procedure. The nurses executed their role with diligence and due care. As for Brian's being discharged before he was able to catheterize himself, this might be explained as a consequence of rigid hospital organizational policies rather than of deficiencies in care from any part of the team.

Following the beneficence model's requirement of doing what is best for the patient, the surgeon could view his actions as directed at fulfilling a primary responsibility to ensure a safe surgical intervention. The problem had been identified; a treatment had been proposed and from a purely technical point of view it had been successful. He could have argued that even though there was reason to suspect underlying psychological problems in the relationship between the mother and the child, these were not sufficiently severe to alter the decision to go ahead with the surgery. In his opinion, the earlier these operations were performed the better, even if there were problems at the beginning.

The surgeon had also to think about his other patients and keeping Brian in hospital necessarily meant that others had to wait for important treatment. Trying to deal equitably with patients and judge when parents were able to take over the responsibility for caring for their children again was always a difficult business but in this case he felt they would be able to manage. Thus, all of these factors being taken into consideration, the best thing for Brian was discharge with follow-up at one of his clinics.

The nursing staff, equally, felt justified in their treatment of Brian. Guided by the emerging patient autonomy model, they had sought to establish a close relationship with Brian and his family. They had identified a number of potential problem areas and were particularly concerned about the mother's feelings of guilt and failure over Brian's condition. These difficulties of the mother's had apparently never been resolved and they were consequently affecting the way mother and son interacted with each other. Brian was often aggressive and rude to her, refusing to comply with her wishes and even doing the opposite of what she asked. The nursing staff had talked to each other about this and had involved the clinical nurse specialist who had helped them devise a programme of activities to help Brian and his mother learn how to do the intermittent catheterization.

They saw the intervention of the surgeon as a necessary part of the restorative process. Their view was that neither Brian nor his mother was ready to go through with this sort of treatment and they had intimated as much – even though only to each other. So, after their initial anger at Brian's discharge, they resigned themselves to the fact, confident in their view that the procedure should not have been undertaken in the first place.

Both groups of professionals therefore could defend their actions on the grounds of doing what was best for the patient, utilizing their skills and knowledge for the welfare of the individuals and acting on what they believed were his best interests. Yet the perspectives were at variance: the surgeon viewed his responsibility in terms of effective surgical technique and conducted his deliberation within a paternalistic model; the nurses, working with the patient autonomy model, began from a social-psychological base and moved into a consideration of the more long-term management problems the boy would face.

It is not possible to accept that both positions are totally justified, not least because the goal of getting Brian independent in his elimination habits had not been achieved at discharge and no concrete plan had been established. This was too central a goal for its non-achievement to be easily discounted. The anger and resentment of the nursing staff also pointed to a problem in communication between themselves and their medical colleagues. This could be explained (within this context) as intransigence on both sides where the surgeon was convinced that he knew what was best for Brian given his position, knowledge and experience, while the nursing staff likewise believed that they had a special monopoly on the correct interpretation of the situation. Because both parties saw themselves as having done what was right, they entered into a stalemate, unwilling (or indeed unable) to enter into dialogue with each other. Given such outcomes we will have to dismiss the first hypothesis and conclude that it is impossible for both parties to sustain the view that their behaviour was right or justified.

5.7 SECOND HYPOTHESIS: DOCTORS RIGHT – NURSES WRONG

This brings us to the next hypothesis. Here it might be thought that the medical interpretation of the case is the more accurate and therefore the nursing position of challenging the medical decision ought to be ignored. This position could draw plausibility from the traditional image of the doctor–nurse relationship which, as we have already noted, is based on a paternalistic–submissive model. In addition to the considerations previously noted in vindication of the doctor, it could also be argued that the problem occurred because nurses chose to take patient care into their own hands and thereby challenge the sound judgement of the doctor. They were not supposed to do this and their protestations were, for the most part, minor inconveniences compared to the overall responsibility carried by the surgeon. The inconvenience caused by some nurses who chose to take the medical decision into their own hands was quite tiresome. Doctors, being more highly trained and having to make numerous decisions about patient welfare in the course of their daily work, are more able to judge what was best for their patients. Nurses do not have equivalent skills or knowledge; they do not have the power to admit or discharge patients, nor do they have to stand accountable for patient care. Their main function is to co-operate with the medical team and keep patients comfortable.

Given this highly traditional and somewhat stereotypical description of a medical perspective on the nature of the doctor–nurse relationship, in Brian's case a strong plea could be made by the surgeon in terms of his autonomous clinical position and the inappropriateness of nursing staff's questioning his practice. Granted that nurses are to be 'obedient servants of a master' (Moore, 1935), their querying the medical decision could be dismissed as a sign of malevolence and unworthiness and need not be acknowledged as a real challenge to the surgeon's clinical credibility. When matters are viewed in this perspective, there appears to be no major problem about Brian's treatment. He had the best care for the length of time required; he would be seen at out-patients' clinic and any minor problems could be dealt with there.

However, this position is unacceptable on a number of counts. First, the nurses' objections to Brian's treatment cannot be ignored on the grounds that nurses should obey doctors. Codes of both medical and nursing ethics stress the responsibility of the professional to use his or her skills and knowledge in the service of mankind and in respecting fellow human beings. Bearing that responsibility is part of the nurse's job. Thus, despite the dominant–submissive nature of the doctor–nurse relationship, the nursing perspective on the patient's welfare has a right to be heard just as the medical voice does.

Second, in Brian's case the nurses had identified a number of deficiencies in previous treatment and had picked up behavioural and psychological problems which they reckoned would obstruct progress towards the overall goal. Either the surgeon had considered these issues and dismissed them or he had not picked them up. What the nursing staff required was some way of opening up the dialogue between themselves and their medical colleagues to explore these issues. Even this would be impossible if the plea envisaged above were to prevail.

Third, even within the purview of the medical beneficence model where the primary objective of the doctor is to do his best for his patient, there could be no justification for ignoring new or different information about the patient. If information was dismissed because it came from a source considered to be unreliable and yet was offering a number of alternative perspectives relating to treatment and care, it would be even more necessary for the doctor to be able to justify on rational grounds his assessment of the information as useless. In every respect it would be incumbent on the doctor to consider the information and make a fair assessment of it.

It appears, then, that the view that there really was no problem with the treatment cannot be sustained. The problem was not one of disrespectful and truculent nurses challenging the better judgement of their superiors. It was more to do with how a doctor learns to accept alternative views about the care and treatment of his patients without dismissing the information as unimportant or discredited in advance. In Brian's case, therefore, because of the clinical evidence amassed by the nurses which identified numerous management problems, the hypothesis that the doctor was justified in his actions and the nurses were wrong is unacceptable.

5.8 THIRD HYPOTHESIS: DOCTORS WRONG – NURSES RIGHT

In support of the third hypothesis it might be argued that the surgeon's judgement was suspect and that he had carried out surgery without fully discussing the underlying problems of the case. There is no evidence that a case conference had been called and that the views and opinions of other professionals had been sought. Little interest had been shown in Brian's catheter management problems, even when the surgeon was informed about them by nursing staff. From this evidence one could conclude that the doctor's actions were more in question than those of the nurse.

The nurses, for their part, had seen their responsibility in terms of engaging with the boy and his mother, had analysed a number of pressing problems and identified the particular nursing issues that had to be addressed. They had also sought specialist advice and support when they became aware of the complex nature of the problem they were dealing with. (This reflects one aspect of many professional codes of conduct where the nurse is enjoined to recognize her own level of competence and seek help when she cannot meet the patient's needs.) They then worked out a treatment plan and agreed a number of patient objectives. Throughout, the nursing staff were acting independently, responsibly, and for the good of the patient.

Failure to achieve the goals set for the patient was the fault of their medical colleague who had discharged Brian against their wishes. They felt justified regarding the care they had given Brian but were angry and frustrated that the surgeon was able to discharge the boy without consulting them. In fact, they reckoned that they had done a very good job in trying to patch up a situation that ought not to have arisen if they had been involved early on in the decision-making process and if the surgeon had been more open to alternative views about what was best for Brian.

It would, however, be erroneous to accept this position as the most satisfactory analysis of the case. If we did we would be overlooking a number of deficiencies in the nurses' conduct regarding how they chose to communicate their intentions to their medical colleagues. We know from the case study that the surgeon had not been kept informed about the nurse's assessment and treatment of Brian's catheter management problems. He did not know of the existence of the clinical nurse specialist and, justifiably, was rather angry that additional experts were being used without his knowledge. The nursing staff may have been technically correct in their judgement of Brian's problem and in treating him but they had committed a number of what Bosk (1979) calls normative errors which undermined their position.

5.9 FOURTH HYPOTHESIS: DOCTORS WRONG – NURSES WRONG

The fourth hypothesis to be considered is that in the management of Brian and his catheter both the medical and the nursing staff bear responsibility for the inadequacies in care. Neither party, according to this hypothesis, was wholly in the right or exclusively to blame. A possibility to be explored in this connection is that a large portion of the problem rests on the ineffective communication between the medical and nursing staff.

The surgeon, it could be argued, had failed to define Brian's problem in broad enough terms. He had chosen to remain within the confines of the somatic medical model and had not wished to explore the dynamics between Brian and his mother. He had not thought through the management and retraining issues of the case and had considered the task purely in terms of surgical intervention. Failure to establish a clear-cut plan of action for chronic problems in surgical patients is a common occurrence and is classed as a judgemental error (Bosk, 1979, p. 48). Bosk quotes a chief resident on this subject:

Surgeons in general don't like theoretical or psychological problems. Things are either black or white. If they don't understand something, they try to put it out of their minds. . . . One of the worst things that can happen to a patient is to spend a long time on a surgical service. Surgeons lose interest in chronic problems

If Mr White was beginning to see Brian's case in this light then he should have asked for consultations from medical colleagues – the child psychiatrist regarding the problem with the mother, the psychologist regarding the retraining regimen – if he did not want to use the expertise of the nurse. His actions could be questioned on at least two counts: if he was not prepared to involve himself in the more long term aspects of the case then he should have recognized the need to establish effective communication with those who would: and if he chose not to discuss the longer term issues with other personnel then he was effectively taking that responsibility upon himself. He was thus making himself accountable for both the short term and the long term care. In discharging Brian before satisfactory outcomes had been secured for some of the longer term objectives, Mr White was making his overall handling of the case suspect.

Being more accustomed to dealing with management problems in general and having to work closely with patients through the numerous phases of recovery and management of illness, the nursing staff had already identified a number of deficiencies in the care being offered to Brian. Their decision not to confront Mr White early on in Brian's treatment and to clarify the boundaries of their respective roles may have accentuated the problems that eventually emerged. Essentially the nursing staff failed to communicate the nursing perspective that they were employing in organizing Brian's care, and by that failure they permitted Mr White to continue harbouring his notion of nurses as doctors' assistants. Whether they had ever tried to present the more autonomous nursing role to him is another question but it would seem from his behaviour that he was in the grip of the traditional understanding of the nurse as helper.

Not only had the nurses failed to communicate information about themselves and their method of organizing their work but they also failed to transmit the concerns they had about Brian plus the additional information they had amassed. They had not documented it or shared it on the consultant's rounds: if they did attempt to share it, it was not received. They had not told the surgeon of the clinical nurse specialist's involvement and her plans to start working with Brian. In all they had adopted a rather negative, defensive approach to their care which manifested itself as a reluctance to share what they were doing with their colleagues.

It may be that this lack of communication arose from frustration and from earlier attempts to enter into dialogue that had been ignored. However, this is not the point. The point is that, for whatever reason, the nursing staff had proceeded to set in motion a series of interventions which, whilst conforming to the overall goal for Brian, were not accepted as legitimate by the surgeon either because he had not been consulted about them or because he felt the nurses were encroaching on his territory.

The nurses' defensive reactions, when challenged by Mr White, did not help the situation. Their resignation to the fact that Brian would after all be discharged, despite what they thought, reinforced their feeling of impotence. It also undermined their right to practise nursing in an independent and professional way.

Interestingly, the doctor's failure to recognize the need for professional support and help derives from the same sources as the nurses' reluctance to communicate more openly about their nursing interventions with patients. Both groups can be seen to be victims of a very rigid but powerful social system that demands independence, autonomy, authority, and unilateral decision-making from surgeons and demands dependent, nonautonomous, submissive behaviour from nurses. The inappropriateness of this system is well illustrated in Brian's case where the boy suffered as a result of the inability of professional colleagues to communicate effectively with each other.

5.10 SOLUTIONS

Essentially, there are five things that could be done to improve the situation. First, a more patient-centred approach to medical care should be rekindled, with doctors acknowledging the reality of multidisciplinary care and the importance of respecting others' contributions, never using a colleague merely as a means to an end, and recognizing and valuing the particular contribution each person plays in improving the quality of care. Second, there should be a greater acceptance of the autonomous role of the nurse and her role in decision-making about patient care. This would change the relationship from one of inequality to one based on mutual respect, partnership and complementarity of roles. Third, for this to happen nurses need to be able to express in clear, unambiguous terms what the nature of their contribution to patient care consists of, how it is documented and what advantages it confers upon the patient. Fourth, related to the greater clarity in describing the nurse's role and function is the need to protect and strengthen her clinical position. This requires the devolution of decision-making about nursing to the level of nurse–patient interaction, the shedding of hierarchical nurse management structures and the development of a number of clinical specialist roles which enhance practice. The final action needed relates to the way doctors and nurses talk to each other. Simpler ways of communicating activities and actions of either group are needed; more effective means of involving various specialities in decision-making processes are required and ways of being able to challenge the decisions and actions of colleagues have to be given serious thought.

The underlying ethical positions that have supported the traditional medical and nursing perspectives on roles and behaviour need also to be reviewed. As we saw in Chapter Four, the traditional medical beneficence model described by Beauchamp and McCullough 1984 requires practitioners who exercise such virtues as truthfulness, trustworthiness, faithfulness and the like (Beauchamp and McCullough, 1984, p. 40). Although the patient is at a disadvantage in relation to the doctor, this can be compensated for by the doctor's exercise of such virtues. Abuse of the beneficence model is thus related to the failure of the medical practitioner to discharge his moral obligation to his patient through virtuous behaviour.

The traditional way of thinking about the doctor–patient relationship involves activity on the doctor's side and passivity on the patient's side. (The very word 'patient' shows its origin in the context of that way of thinking.) But there is scope for rethinking that relationship, and some rethinking is already occurring. Szasz and Hollender's (1956) model of medical intervention offers legitimate alternatives to the active–passive image of the doctor–patient relationship. Concepts such as negotiation, partnership and dialogue increasingly find a home in medical thinking, particularly in the emerging patient–autonomy model of practice.

How such changes affect the practitioner's view of himself and his notion of how others view him is extremely important, particularly in connection with the doctor–nurse relationship. The nurse too has undergone many changes and has to cope with several areas of conflict in her perception of her role. She may be unclear whether she should conform to the traditional obedience model, seductive as it is in terms of the gender stereotyping, the hierarchical nursing system and the uniforms, all of which provide security to the neophyte nurse. Or she may opt for the contemporary nurse-as-autonomous-practitioner and so-called champion of patients' rights, and be besieged by the legion of contradictions existing in nursing practice. She is exhorted to be the patient's advocate and finds that she, like the patient, is relatively invisible when it comes to challenging medical decisions. She may decide to defend her right to practice nursing only to find that her rights are overruled by other authorities. Yarling and McElmurry (1986) think that the only real solution to this problem is for nurses to become independent practitioners, employed like their medical colleagues on a contractual basis by hospitals. A more appealing (and less militant) solution might be a shift in the focus of accountability from other health care professionals to the patients themselves. This would fit with the nursing notion that health care should be based more on a patient autonomy model than a beneficence model.

Such proposals will be useful to the extent that changes in the established way of thinking about how doctors and nurses give care can improve the patient's experience of health care interventions. Common complaints continue to be linked to patients feeling uninvolved with, uninformed about, and dissociated from much of what is happening to them. This may suggest that part of our professional training immunizes us against such realities and makes us prey to the belief that we know better than people themselves what is good for them and to the rhetoric associated with that belief.

How we reach the point of offering doctors and nurses more flexibility in the roles they undertake, how we achieve collaborative teamwork, and how we meet the ever increasing demand for medical and nursing care are major issues. Some advantages must be obtained from giving patients more responsibility for their own health and aiming to provide them (and their carers) with elementary knowledge about healthy living. Such an approach could be highly effective in improving health care services, given changes in traditional roles and a more imaginative approach to medical and nursing education. In order for doctor–nurse relationships to flourish there must be more collaboration during training, where mutual trust and respect are built up and where the scientific and ethical principles of either professional can be explored in the safety of the lecture theatre and the seminar room.

There should be more emphasis on patient autonomy and its implications for the physician's role. Joint research and evaluation projects could also help to elucidate the complementary relations of both professions. This would consolidate awareness of the need for partnership and effective communication between groups and identify how best to achieve it. Ultimately what is required to benefit the patient is a team of doctors and nurses who can agree on shared objectives for care and who can communicate effectively with each other on how these can best be achieved. In this perspective there is no room for rudeness or forcing others to compromise their values for the sake of a colleague.

5.11 CONCLUSION

In this chapter we have identified some pervasive problems and have seen that solutions are not to be found easily and are not to be found only at the level of interaction between individuals. We have indicated some ways in which there could be movement towards solutions and we have highlighted the need for future work and the character of that work.

SIX

Private: don't intrude

6.1 CONFIDENTIALITY

By common consent, confidentiality is an important element in the ethics of nursing. Sometimes there is said to be a *duty* or *obligation* of confidentiality. Codes of ethics for nurses normally include reference to confidentiality. Sometimes confidentiality is spoken of as a fundamental *right* of persons receiving health care. It is repeatedly stressed that patients' or clients' preference for keeping personal information secret should be respected. Normally, according to the standard view, nurses and others should act against that preference only to the extent that acting against it is necessary for the care of the person. That is to say, in the normal way of things disclosing confidential information against a patient's wishes would need to be justified as an instance of justifiable paternalism (see Chapter Three above). Exceptionally, it is usually suggested, health care workers may act against the preference for the sake of important matters of public interest or the interest of other individuals. Examples of this are considered in section 6.6, below.

The nurse who is at ease with her work will be sensitive to features of a situation that relate to confidentiality and privacy. She will be quick to pick up signs of a patient's not realizing that information is passed about within the health care team. She will likewise be quick to spot the potential for breach of confidence in any corner-cutting practices that have grown up.

In section 6.2 we try to say more exactly what confidentiality is and what it means to say that there is a duty or obligation of confidentiality and to say that people have a right to it. Later, in section 6.7, we consider more fully the virtue that makes a person readily able to handle matters of confidentiality well.

6.2 WHAT IS CONFIDENTIALITY?

There are things about everyone that are not generally known. Some things about a person are known, in the normal course of events, only to friends or family; some might not be known to anyone at all apart from the person herself or himself. Sometimes a person discloses such things to another who would not in the normal course of events have had access to them, the disclosure being made on the understanding – or with the request – that what is disclosed will be kept restricted.

Wherever there is confidentiality, there is a request or understanding concerning the limits of further disclosure. Confidentiality is said to be *breached* if confidential information is disclosed beyond those limits. We could put this another way by saying that there is always a *circle of confidentiality* consisting of those people with whom the confidential information can be shared without breach of confidentiality. To know exactly what confidentiality involves in a particular case is to know what the limits of the circle are. In some cases what is requested or understood is that there is to be no further disclosure at all; then the circle of confidentiality is just the one person to whom the information was confided. In other cases further disclosure is to be restricted to a particular group of people; that group is then the circle of confidentiality. 'Don't tell any grown-ups' permits the information to be passed on to children but not to adults.

Maintaining confidentiality is a matter of behaving in such a way as not to bring about a breach of confidentiality. If something has been revealed to me in confidence and I disclose it to someone else in the circle of confidentiality, maintaining confidentiality involves my ensuring that that other person will not disclose the information outside the circle of confidentiality.

Often the circle of confidentiality will be just those people who are directly involved in the care and treatment of the person concerned. Sometimes information may be confided in the nurse as an individual, so that she alone is in the circle of confidentiality. If the information – perhaps about domestic circumstances or relations with a spouse – strikes the nurse as relevant to the care of the patient, she may ask the patient to extend the circle of confidentiality to include the health care team. Thus the circle of confidentiality may be fixed as a result of an initiative made by the nurse.

In section 6.1 there was talk of a duty and a right of confidentiality. We are now in a position to explain that talk. To say that there is a moral *duty* or *obligation* of confidentiality is to say that a person – or circle of persons – to whom such things are disclosed ought not to disclose them further except within the relevant limits. To say that there is a moral *right* to confidentiality is to say that a person who has disclosed something to another in confidence would be wronged if that other were then to disclose it beyond the relevant limits.

6.3 WHY CONFIDENTIALITY MATTERS

Confidentiality in health care is important for a number of reasons. One reason – a utilitarian reason – is based on the fact that confidentiality is something that people in general seem to want. There are also non-utilitarian reasons: that personal information is a kind of personal property, that confidentiality is a matter of decency, that confidentiality is important because privacy is important, and that confidentiality is a matter of respecting persons. Here we shall develop these reasons, especially the connection with privacy. Later we shall consider some difficult cases in the light of the reasons discussed here.

Consequences of confidentiality

Consider first the utilitarian reason. It is that confidentiality is important because the practice of keeping personal information about patients and clients secret has good consequences (see section 2.5, above). Because people in fact want personal information about themselves kept confidential and do not like highly personal information about themselves to be bandied about, made available to strangers, and made the subject of gossip – because of all this the practice of keeping such information secret makes people more likely to present themselves for health care when they need it and more likely to be open in giving health care professionals necessary information.

Information as property

A second reason involves the idea that personal information is a kind of property. Suppose Alice lends Beth a watch. There are things that Beth could permissibly do with her own watch which she could not do with Alice's; for example, she could permissibly lend out her own watch – but not Alice's – to someone else. Again, Alice might invite Beth into her home to baby-sit; there are things that Beth ought not to do with Alice's home (taking down the wallpaper, for example, or bringing a dozen friends round) which it would be perfectly all right for her to do with her own. In the same way, the argument goes, information of a personal kind about Alice is Alice's information, and Beth is not at liberty to treat it as though it were her own. The right to personal property is regarded by many as a fundamental human right. Confidentiality is important because intimate information about oneself is an especially personal kind of property.

Confidentiality as decency

A third reason is that, in any society, there are certain things that should be kept quiet and, as a matter of decency, should not be made public and noised abroad. What people see as matters of decency varies from culture to culture; but, whatever a patient's cultural background, there will be facts about the patient which are covered by their culture's concept of decency. Such information is likely to be among the things that a nurse comes to know in the course of making a nursing assessment, giving care and communicating with colleagues. Maintaining confidentiality is important because it is the prevention of the indecent exposure of private information. What is intimate should remain intimate and not become the currency of the market place – even the localized market place, like the staff canteen.

Confidentiality as privacy

A fourth reason for the importance of confidentiality is that maintaining confidentiality is a way of protecting a person's privacy. Privacy in turn is important because there is a profound human need for it. Some philosophers have argued, moreover, that having some control of whether one's thoughts, feelings and personal information are revealed or concealed is necessary for selfhood and for tolerable interpersonal relations (cf. Fried, 1984; Benn, 1984; Gerstein, 1984; Marshall, 1988).

Confidentiality as respecting persons

A fifth reason concerns respect for persons. Other people's life plans are to be respected. Personal autonomy centrally involves having one's own plans, projects, ambitions, etc. Autonomous persons have their own views as to how their own lives are to develop and as to what is to have an important place in those lives. To respect a person's autonomy is to treat the person as having a right to determine what is for them more important and less important. It is to treat them as having a right to determine – within suitable limits – how to live their life. For each of us there are things which are private or secret. A person's choice of a way of living includes choices about what is more secret or private and what is less so. Respecting a person's autonomy involves respecting those choices and hence having reason to treat as intimate and private those things that, in the person's chosen way of living, are intimate and private.

In accepting information as confidential, one makes one's own the other's decision against further disclosure. Although one may see reason to impart it further and may seek to persuade the imparter to agree to that, her or his actual decision is what one accepts as settling the matter. In doing this one is respecting the person's project concerning her or his intimate information – and perhaps respecting her or his judgement/ decision as to what is in the relevant way intimate. Here, respecting someone's judgement or decision would be treating it as final. Confidentiality is important as a way of respecting people's life plans.

In this section we have noted various reasons for holding that confidentiality matters. Feelings are sometimes good indicators of things mattering to a person. Felt distress on discovering that one's personal information has been spread around indicates that secrecy matters to one and indicates how much it matters. Some discussions tacitly assume that breaches of privacy and confidentiality are undesirable because they cause distress. But this is only a part of the story. In the main they cause distress because they are undesirable and they are undesirable for reasons like the ones given above. The fact – if it is a fact – that breaches of privacy and confidentiality cause distress is not the only reason for maintaining privacy and confidentiality.

6.4 PRIVATE AND PUBLIC SPACES

Some things about a person are ordinarily known only to that person. Some are known to immediate family, some to long-standing friends, some to casual acquaintances, some to anyone who cares to find out. We could think of all the information about a person as being distributed in a collection of different spaces. There is a most intimate space within which are the person's most secret thoughts, feelings, hopes, fears, etc. Only the person herself/himself has ready access to this space. There is a less private space housing the things about the person that those people to whom she is the closest have ready access – perhaps some members of her family, perhaps some very close friends. A wider space holds the information to which the rest of the family has access. There is a still wider one to which long-standing acquaintances (colleagues at work, members of the same church, tennis club, etc.) have access, and yet another space to which more casual acquaintances have access. The widest space is the public domain.

Some of these spaces are inside others. Sometimes two spaces overlap without either being entirely within the other. (Dramatic cases of people living 'double lives' – perhaps with two families each of which is unaware of the other's existence – are of this kind. Less dramatic cases are common; there is often a 'side' of a person which is to be seen only in the home and another 'side' which is known only to workmates.)

Each person has a collection of such spaces. Confidentiality arises when a person admits to one of the more private spaces some other person or group. The circle of confidentiality is that group of people who are given access to information in a space to which they would ordinarily not have access.

The suggestion in the last section that confidentiality is a matter of decency involves the idea that the whereabouts in this system of spaces of certain information is not for the individual to determine but is fixed by norms transcending the individual. On this view, if the individual moves into a wider space what belongs in a narrower one, the individual is committing an impropriety akin to indecent exposure.

Again, which information and which facets of a person's character are to go into which space is part of what goes into a way of living a life. Respecting persons involves respecting their life plans and hence their location of information in one space rather than another. This way of respecting persons concerns not only the transmitting of information but also attitudes. Making a person's private space a subject of mocking laughter with friends even without the disclosure of confidential information is contrary to the spirit of confidentiality.

Confidentiality permits private things to be spoken of between persons without thereby becoming public. It provides something intermediate between two extremes – the extreme of *total secrecy* (something locked in my own breast) and the extreme of *total access* (something which is out in the open – in the public domain – and can be perused by anyone who takes the trouble to seek it out).

6.5 DELIBERATING ABOUT CONFIDENTIALITY

We noted earlier that moral deliberation involves an appreciation of the agent's situation, one or more principles, a review of possible courses of action, and a decision. Deliberation can be instantaneous and so much a matter of routine as to be almost unconscious. For example, the situation may be that a nurse is sitting with well-liked colleagues in the canteen, and a light-hearted conversation has reached a point at which an anecdote about one of the current patients would be especially amusing. Recounting the anecdote would be a possible course of action. However, the nurse immediately notes that that particular anecdote would involve disclosing personal information about the patient. This brings the principle of confidentiality into play, a principle which is now second nature to the nurse. She reflects that disclosing the information here would have no bearing on care of the patient. She then decides not to regale her friends with that story. (Or perhaps the story is *so* amusing that she decides to tell it anyway. Deliberation does not always issue in morally correct decisions.)

Often a major concern in the nurse's deliberation will be the concern to find a morally correct decision or the morally best defensible decision. In many cases there will be no real difficulty in arriving at such a decision (although some firmness might occasionally be needed to stick to it in the face of a persistent, cunning or bullying enquirer). For example, if a patient is in hospital for a third pregnancy termination, other patients should not be told about that patient's previous terminations; a casual enquirer should not be told a patient's diagnosis; a health visitor should not gossip in one home about the client in another. In cases like these, the fact that the disclosure of confidential information is being requested will be salient in the situation as the nurse sees it. The principle of confidentiality will be called into play at once. No weighty considerations favouring disclosure are to hand. So only courses of action involving refusal to breach confidentiality will feature as serious options.

Among the factors that may feature in an appreciation of a situation in the context of deliberation about confidentiality are the status of a piece of information (is it confidential or not?) and the circle of confidentiality (did the patient mean this information not to reach a visiting cousin?). Appreciating the situation may not be a trivial task. If the information is personal and non-clinical in character it may be information of a kind that some people prefer to keep secret and others do not; and it may have been made known to the nurse in a context of at most implied confidentiality. Again, a patient's wish to keep certain information within the family might leave the nurse in doubt as to whether immediate or extended family is meant. It is clearly not possible to eliminate all such unclarity from ordinary communication. The scope for error in situation-appreciation is just something that people have to live with and make the best of.

Again, some self-knowledge may be in order. If one is secretive and tight-lipped by nature, one needs to be on guard against too hastily assuming that a certain person is outside the circle of confidentiality. If, on the other hand, one is a relaxed and open person who generally lets information flow freely, one needs to take care that one has not overlooked a patient's tacit request for discretion (a request that might be the easier to overlook since one would never have made it oneself).

Where there is good reason to disclose information beyond the circle of confidentiality, there may be opportunity to obtain the patient's consent to its disclosure. The patient has the power to widen the circle of confidentiality, and this is what happens when uncoerced consent is given. If consent cannot be obtained, there will be more of a problem.

One type of situation is envisaged in section 3 of the RCN's *Guidelines on Confidentiality in Nursing* (1980). This is the situation where the relatives of a client or patient ask the nurse for information which she holds in confidence. The nurse's appreciation of the situation will take in facts (the information she has about the patient, the fact that the relatives have asked for some information, how closely related they are to the patient, whatever she knows about the preferences of the patient – the patient may have expressed resentment of the nosiness of some relatives – and about how well they get on), it will take in who the parties are (apart from the patient and the relatives and the nurse herself, perhaps other relatives, friends, and other members of the health care team need to be taken into account) and what their interests, needs, and rights are.

The RCN guidelines note that the nurse must decide what is in the best interest of the patient or client. However, we should note that this may not decide the matter. Suppose that, although the patient has not given consent, the nurse is in no doubt, on reflection, that it is in the best interest of the patient or client for the information to be conveyed to the relatives. This alone is not sufficient ground for the nurse to pass on the information. It is not just a question of the patient's interests. The patient's plans for his/her life are also important. This is one of the reasons for the importance of confidentiality. Communicating some nonconfidential information to another party may be the right thing to do when it is in a patient's interest. In the case of confidential information, confidentiality counts for something and the considerations of the patient's interest have to be that much more weighty to outweigh it.

Another consideration that might, on occasion, tip the balance in favour of telling the relatives is consideration of the needs of those relatives themselves (RCN *Guidelines*, 1980, section 3.3.) Suppose the nurse is considering whether this is so in the present case. Then she has to consider not only whether the needs of the relatives outweigh the needs of the patient/client but whether the needs of the relatives outweigh the obligation of confidentiality. The bond of confidentiality is something over and above the needs of the patient, and it is that bond which must be superseded or outweighed if disclosing the information is to be justified.

If one is to deliberate well about questions of confidentiality, one needs to be aware that confidentiality is a further consideration over and above the needs of the people involved. So, when deliberating in a situation where two of the options are to keep confidence and to breach confidence by disclosing information to the relatives, the deliberating nurse needs to ask herself not only 'Are the needs of the relatives here greater than those of the patient?' but also 'Despite the strength of the bond of confidentiality, are the needs of the relatives here sufficient to supersede that bond?'

If only the first question is asked, then confidentiality is treated as counting for nothing.

Tate gives the example of a young woman hospital patient with uterine bleeding who tells a student nurse in confidence that she is pregnant and has attempted to bring about an abortion. She stresses that she does not want the doctor to know. The nurse then tells the doctor who, by asking the patient well-judged questions, gets the patient to tell him everything without the nurse's breach of confidence being revealed (see Tate, 1977, p. 21).

Without knowing the full details of the case outlined, let us imaginatively consider how the student nurse might have deliberated. The nurse's appreciation of the situation, after she has been told of the attempt to bring about an abortion, takes in the stated wishes of the patient, the duty of confidentiality, the interest of the patient, the need for relevant medical information to be available to the health care team. There are at least two possible courses of action. One is to keep secret the confidential information and act as though accepting the patient's stated explanation that such bleeding has occurred several times over a year in connection with her monthly period. The other course is to disclose the information given to her privately by the patient. The nurse concludes that the need for the patient to have appropriate treatment outweighs the duty of confidentiality. Accordingly she decides on disclosure.

Once the doctor is informed, there is another problem. A decision has to be reached as to whether the patient will or will not be told of the breach of confidence. If she is told, it may confirm her in a bitter, cynical mistrust of health care professionals and of people in general; this in turn may make the task of giving her good health care harder. It will also cause distress to the nurse. If, on the other hand, the patient can be brought to disclose the true situation to the doctor, it will be just as though there had been no breach of confidence, and she will get the treatment she needs. The doctor takes this last option and successfully brings it off.

On the face of it, the moral balance sheet here will include the following. On the credit side are the eventual openness of communication between the patient and the doctor, the securing of appropriate treatment for the patient, the avoidance of bitterness in the patient, the avoidance of distress to the nurse; on the debit side are the nurse's breach of confidence and the doctor's lack of candour in manipulating the patient into disclosing the true story. The outcome seems to be the least unsatisfactory one. The credits are in the main evaluative: a good state of affairs is brought about. The debits are of other kinds: acts of a kind that one ordinarily ought not to do – acts of breaking confidence and deceitful concealment – are done. This does not appear to be a case of value outweighing rights and duties. It is not that, because of her medical needs, the patient has no right to confidentiality. It is rather that, despite the right to confidentiality that she has, her medical need is the most important factor.

However, there are other possible ways of interpreting the situation. It may be that at a deeper level the patient was seeking the assistance of the nurse and doctor in making it easier for her to tell the doctor what he needed to know. In that case, in telling the doctor, the nurse was doing what she had implicitly been asked to do. (The patient surely cannot seriously have expected the nurse to keep the information to herself.) What this possibility brings out is that arriving at an appropriate appreciation of the situation may be not at all a trivial task; either the status of the information or the intended circle of confidentiality may be not what it appears to be.

6.6 SOME CASES

In many cases confidentiality is in conflict with other considerations. Sometimes it may be clear that the other considerations should prevail. Where there are sufficiently important considerations of the public interest (e.g. that a public transport driver has a condition that could lead to a serious accident) or of the rights or welfare of a third party (e.g. a child at risk of sexual or physical abuse) or even the fundamental interests of the person to whom confidentiality is owed, there may be no significant doubt that a way should be found of disclosing confidential information (cf. Walters in Mappes and Zembaty, 1981, pp. 117–118; Muyskens, 1982, pp. 149–153). But there are other cases where considerations of these kinds are less weighty or where considerations of other kinds come into play. In some such cases people find themselves coming to clear moral conclusions, but different people's conclusions conflict with one another. (Thus, some doctors think that the authorities should be notified of indications that a patient is an illegal immigrant, while other doctors are equally clear that this should not be done; see Phillips and Dawson, 1985, pp. 129–131. Again, in the 30.9.88 episode of the British television series 'Casualty' a charge nurse reported to the police a patient admitted with packets of narcotics which she had smuggled into the UK by swallowing them; in that case the script had the doctor first insist that confidentiality was decisive but later come round to the charge nurse's view.) And in other cases people agree in finding it hard to see what should be done.

One well-known disputed case is the Tarasoff case. In October 1969, a man killed a woman two weeks after informing his psychotherapist of his intention to do so. The psychotherapist had not warned the victim or her family. The California Supreme Court's finding was, in effect, that he should have done so (see Tobriner in Mappes and Zembaty, 1981). But there is an important utilitarian argument to the effect that confidentiality should be decisive even in a case of that kind (see Clark in Mappes and Zembaty, 1981; Bok, 1984 and other references given there). The utilitarian argument can be expressed like this. Disclosing the patient's avowed intention would undermine the assurance of confidentiality for those requiring psychiatric attention and would thus lead to more of them remaining untreated, including ones who would be likely to commit acts of violence. In short, the argument is that, although breaching confidentiality in a particular case may save the life of one potential victim, it would lead to greater loss of life on balance. To put it another way, the saving of the lives of potential victims of violent patients is a benefit, the loss of life through confidentiality is a cost, and the cost is worth paying because it is outweighed by the benefit.

This argument states the first of the reasons for the importance of confidentiality set out in section 6.3. It is interesting to consider a case like this in the light of the other reasons. The other reasons were these:

1. personal information is a kind of property,
2. confidentiality is a matter of decency,
3. confidentiality is a matter of privacy, and
4. confidentiality is a matter of respecting persons.

None of these other reasons applies in this case. Consider reason 1. The fact that a hand grenade was my property would not be good reason to leave me murderously in possession of it; so the fact that a murderous intention is my own is similarly not a good reason for others to keep silent about it. Reason 2 has to do with decency, but there is nothing indecent about warning an intended murder victim. Reason 3 concerns privacy; but, while it might be argued that my indulging in daydreams of slaughter is my own private affair, an intention to perform a real killing in the real world is no longer my own private affair. Finally, reason 4 for the importance of confidentiality is respect for a person's right to determine – within suitable limits – how to live her or his life; but it is plain that the choice of a life that includes taking the life of another is not within the suitable limits – and that choice of a life does not have to be respected.

In short, the only considerations that apply in the case outlined are utilitarian ones. The other reasons for the importance of confidentiality do not get a grip. This does not mean that controversy over such a case is easy to settle; but some kinds of moral complexity can be excluded.

Perhaps the same can be said concerning confidentiality and drug smugglers. In their case maintaining confidentiality may obstruct justice and worsen the prospects for those at risk from drug abuse. These are plainly costs. The question arises whether these costs are worth paying for the sake of the benefits of confidentiality in general. The answer may be yes, but only if confidentiality for drug smugglers is inseparable from confidentiality in general. If confidentiality for drug smugglers can be separated from confidentiality in general, then the benefits of confidentiality in general can be had without the costs of extending confidentiality to drug smugglers. Another possibility may be that using confidentiality to protect a drug smuggler is an *abuse* of confidentiality and, in consequence, also a threat to confidentiality (by nourishing the suspicion that confidentiality is not such a good thing after all). If this could be shown then there would be a case for withholding the protection of confidentiality for the sake of confidentiality itself.

6.7 THE VIRTUE OF DISCRETION

A person who has been told by her teachers and by others whose instructions she wishes to follow that confidential information is to be disclosed only for the gravest of reasons can make it her business always to comply with this instruction. A person who is convinced by the moral arguments for a principle of confidentiality can make sure that her conduct is duly guided by that principle. Thus a person may be guided by the principle of confidentiality either from a sense of duty (or loyalty or obedience) or from conviction. She will fight against the inclination to gossip; she will resist the temptation to say 'I shouldn't be telling you this but . . .'. She may occasionally let something confidential slip out; she may unwittingly give things away to someone who is clever at tricking people into disclosing things; she may reluctantly and uneasily let someone have access to information when they have confused her with a mass of arguments which she could not quite follow but which sounded pretty plausible. But in the main she will not knowingly disclose confidential information without very good reason.

However, her handling of problems of confidentiality would be more surely founded if it stemmed not just from what she had been told to do and not just from her being convinced by a carefully argued case but from the kind of person she is. Let us try to characterize the kind of person to whom it comes naturally to handle matters of confidentiality well; in other words let us characterize the virtue which would make someone able to handle matters of confidentiality well.

Common language seems not to have a name for this virtue. Sissela Bok (1984) has suggested taking the existing word 'discretion' and using it to stand for the virtue in question. That is what we shall do here. In this book, then, **discretion** is to be understood as the virtue of coping well with confidentiality, secrecy and privacy.

Virtue is in part a matter of habits of conduct. The habits that a person with the virtue of discretion will have are communicative habits. A discreet person will not be in the habit of impulsively saying whatever happens to be uppermost in her mind at the time. Her preferred forms of entertainment will tend not to include trading juicy pieces of information about people who would prefer the information not to circulate. (No doubt she will enjoy harmless gossip as much as the next person, but she will be sensitive to the limits and to the area where humour shades off into malice.) Equally she will not be in the habit of eavesdropping. And, while being a good listener, she will not be in the habit of using listening skills to simulate an attitude of caring or attentively to ease another into more self-disclosure than that other needs or wants to make. In addition to behavioural habits, there are mental habits. Very often something is disclosed only because the speaker had not given any thought to whether it was confidential or not. A discreet person will tend not to make this mistake. She will have the mental habit of locating each new piece of information that comes her way in its appropriate circle of confidentiality. Thus who it can be appropriately passed on to is something that she will have considered long before there is any occasion for passing it on to anyone at all. It is to be stressed that, for the discreet person, this will not be a mental effort made each time something new is learned. It is rather something that will occur effortlessly. She will no doubt acknowledge that in some situations confidentiality has to be broken. But among her habits will be some which make situations less likely to arise.

As well as habits, virtues characteristically involve certain concerns. A discreet person cares about privacy, decency and the like. She will care that private and intimate things not be made public. Having this concern is not the same as being incurious. The discreet person may be as curious as anyone else about what someone else does or daydreams about in private; but her concern that private things remain private will make her disinclined to pry or spy or eavesdrop even if she is curious and has the opportunity.

A concern for one's own privacy is inseparable from the concern for the privacy of others. Sissela Bok (1984, p. 21; cf. p. 46) goes so far as to speak of sacredness in this connection.

> Without perceiving some sacredness in human identity, individuals are out of touch with the depth they might feel in themselves and respond to in others. Given such a sense, however, certain intrusions are felt as violations – a few even as desecrations.

The discreet person's concern for privacy will not be restricted to adults or peers but will embrace the privacy of the disadvantaged, children and patients (cf. Bok, 1984, p. 43). Her concern for confidentiality is a concern that confidential things not go further than they should. Her concern is not just that *she* get things right, but that they are got right by others as well; thus it includes a concern that record keeping systems not be leaky and that other people with access to the records also respect confidentiality (see UKCC, 1987, sections C 2 and C 3). She will also tend to have feelings of certain kinds. She will feel uneasiness or distress if intimate information is bandied about in her presence, or if colleagues talk in a way that suggests that privacy does not matter. In a situation where there is no doubt that disclosing confidential information is what ought to be done, she will still feel compunction at disclosing it.

There is a very great deal to be said about the cognitive side of discretion. This is prominent in the RCN's *Guidelines on Confidentiality in Nursing*, 1980. In section 7.4 it is noted that 'student nurses should be encouraged to develop a sensitivity to confidential information'. Such a sensitivity is discussed by Sissela Bok:

> At its best, discretion is the intuitive ability to discern what is and is not intrusive and injurious, and to use this discernment in responding to the conflicts everyone experiences as insider and outsider. It is an acquired capacity to navigate in and between the worlds of personal and shared experience, coping with the moral questions about what is fair or unfair, truthful or deceptive, helpful or harmful.
>
> (Bok, 1984, p. 41)

Communicative judgement is important:

> . . . a nurse must be aware of the patient's/client's expectations of her and appreciate that everything the patient/client tells her is not necessarily information to be passed to others. On the other hand, the nurse may be the recipient of information which the patient/client wishes his/ her doctor to know but does not feel able to communicate it directly. The nurse should be able to ascertain if such is the case by further questioning of the patient/client.
>
> (Royal College of Nursing, 1980, section 2–1)

This has to do with the cognitive dimension of discretion. Whereas in the ideally explicit case one party will ask for a certain piece of information to be kept confidential, in many cases that party means it to be understood that the information will be kept confidential but does not actually say so; and in many cases that party means it to be understood which information is to be kept confidential, but does not say which is to be kept confidential and which need not be. To be good in matters of confidentiality, a person needs to have or to cultivate a sensitivity to the implicit intentions of others; she needs to pick up the small signs that what is coming is not for public consumption, and the other small signs that what the patient is now saying is something the patient wants known to others in the health care team. Of course, if in doubt she can always ask – as the RCN 1980 guideline 2.1 suggests. But she is very likely not even to be in doubt unless she has picked up a sign – a gesture, a look, a subtle change in the patient's voice – which prompts her to wonder whether this is something the patient wants to keep secret or whether it is something the patient wants the doctor to know or whether the patient does not mind who knows it.

The cognitive dimension of discretion is involved also in the sensitivity to possible embarrassment of a patient 'in a large open reception or waiting area' (RCN, 1980, section 2.5) being asked to give personal information. For many people it would be very easy simply to overlook that this could be embarrassing for the patient, even though, once it is pointed out to them, they would be concerned about the patient's feelings. A person who has the virtue of discretion will by and large not need to have it pointed out to them.

The cognitive dimension is also involved in connection with accidental disclosure of confidential information. Just as a safety officer instantly spots the potentiality for domestic accidents in a kitchen or living room, so a person with the virtue of discretion will be alive to the scope for accidental disclosure in a situation; she will be quick to remember that someone present is not a member of the team, and quick to notice that the information can be overheard or that someone has not realized that it is confidential, or that it can be overheard. (See RCN, 1980, section 2.7)

The upshot of all this is that for the person with the virtue we are calling discretion it will come naturally to notice, do, feel, and care about things which most of us can notice, do, feel, and care about only erratically and with an effort. Most people will have the virtue at most imperfectly. Even people who have the virtue to a high degree will have off days and even off years. But it does no harm to reflect on what we would ideally wish to be like, or to reflect on what it is that we find so impressive about the colleagues we most admire.

6.8 CONCLUSION

It is important to remember that confidentiality matters. Sometimes discussion of confidentiality degenerates into bluster because, while people sense *that* it matters, they have no articulate idea of *why* it matters. In this chapter we have sought to give a clear account of what confidentiality is and to articulate and explore reasons for thinking that it matters. We have sought also to examine the factors entering into deliberation about problems of confidentiality, and to develop an understanding of the character traits that tend to make a person good at coping with issues of confidentiality.

SEVEN

To tell the truth?

7.1 TRUTH AND AUTONOMY

Why is truth important? One reason is this: having access to true information about matters concerning oneself is important because of its intimate connection with autonomy and agency. Agency is the ability to act. Individual persons are agents; groups of people can also be agents. But the agency of a person or a group can be impaired or diminished. (In section 5.3 above we noted the suggestion that the medical assistant role diminishes the nurse's agency.)

Consider first the autonomy of individuals. When we think of persons being autonomous we think of them being active rather than passive and we think of them as having plans and making decisions. All this involves their being able to deliberate, i.e. to take account of factual information, take note of different possible courses of action, and relate important practical concerns to the information and the alternatives (see section 2.2). A special dignity is attached to taking a hand in shaping events – especially events which are particularly connected with oneself – rather than passively letting things happen to oneself and around oneself. This is reflected in the acute sense of loss often experienced by people who were active but are no longer so.

This special dignity is threatened or undermined if the character of one's actions is not what one takes it to be, or one's plans and decisions are made in the light of wrong information. Ignorance of material information subverts one's acting and one's longer term planning (see section 4.8 above, and Bok, 1980, pp. 18–20). When others keep such information from a person, they are subverting that person's autonomy.

For patients among others, to be given false information about impor-

tant events in their lives is to be rendered powerless and to be deprived
of their autonomy.

(Schröck, 1980, p. 140)

Secondly, consider group autonomy. Often an individual deliberates, plans
and acts as an individual. However, we also co-deliberate, co-plan and
co-act with one another, especially with those persons with whom we have
personal relations. A group of people can be a deliberating, acting and
planning agent; like an individual, it can be autonomous. But its autonomy
is impaired if material information is unavailable to the group; and its
autonomy is also impaired if material information is available to one
member of the group and not to another. Co-deliberation involves the
deliberators having equal access to information which is material to their
deliberation. For example, our deliberation as to whether to go for a
picnic is subverted if I have heard the weather forecast and I withhold
from you the material information that it contained.

The relation between autonomy and truth can be seen in connection
with informed consent. It is widely acknowledged that consent is important. But *why* is it important? It is hard to see why importance should be
ascribed to consent as an ethical matter (rather than just as a matter
of legal defensiveness) unless there is an underlying assumption of the
importance of autonomy. Granted the importance of autonomy, it
becomes important that patients have as much of a hand in their management as possible. And for this they need to be informed.

Morally speaking, then, the point of aiming to get patients' informed
consent comes from the principle of autonomy. By consenting to some
procedure or treatment, a patient makes that procedure or treatment part
of his or her plan. Respecting a person's (possibly imperfect) autonomy
involves thinking that it matters whether what happens to them is part of
their plan or not. But it is important that consent be not just blind consent
but *informed* consent, in other words that the patient understands what
is being consented to. If they consent without understanding at all what
is going to happen to them then their plan has an area of indeterminacy
in it (like a bus timetable where one of the entries says 'mystery tour'
instead of giving route details). With that indeterminacy, the plan would
reflect a lower degree of autonomy. The better the patient's grasp of the
important features of what is going to happen to them, the closer their
consent comes to making the procedure or treatment consistent with
continuing autonomy. Thus, for the same reason that consent is important,
it is also important that patients have true information about what they
are consenting to. False information, poorly understood information and
missing information impair the personal autonomy of the patient.

Informed consent relates also to group autonomy. To the extent that the patient's consent is a significant factor in determining whether a procedure or treatment goes ahead, or even in choosing it, the patient is a co-deliberator along with the professionals in the health care team. Respecting patient autonomy by seeking the active involvement of the patient in her or his own care (see section 4.10 above) is seeking to approximate to a situation where the patient is a full member of the treatment team and care team, so that patient and professionals together constitute a group agent. The autonomy of that agent is undermined if material information is not equally available among its members.

In the case of individual persons and that of groups of persons, truth matters because of its connection with autonomy and agency.

It is worth recalling at this point Virginia Henderson's (1966) well-known statement of the function of nursing:

> The unique function of the nurse is to assist the individual, sick or well, in the performance of those activities contributing to health or its recovery (or to peaceful death) that he would perform unaided if he had the necessary strength, will or knowledge. And to do this in such a way as to help him gain independence as rapidly as possible.

Many other writers have stressed that nursing is concerned with the entire person cared for and that a central aim of nursing care is to bring the person cared for to as complete a degree of autonomy as is possible. Thus it seems agreed that nursing is about restoring individuals as far as is possible to full membership of a community or society of persons who are each in control of their own lives. It is in keeping with this aim not only, where possible, to comply with the wishes of those who want to know how they stand but also to encourage those who do not want to know where they stand towards a more self-possessed position. As well as respecting autonomy where it is present, it is part of the aim of nursing to promote autonomy.

7.2 TRUTH AND ADVANTAGE

The amount of information one obtains for oneself is pretty small. The overwhelming greatest part of the information at a person's disposal has come from sources which the person takes to be reliable. The advantages of such trust over cautious scepticism are immense, as long as the trust does not turn out to be mistaken. Just because it is a matter of taking things for granted, the benefits of trust tend to be invisible most of the time. (When your watch stops you discover how much it was doing for you while it was working normally.)

So one reason for the importance of truthfulness is that it enables people to have confidence in a far wider range of information that they could obtain and check for themselves. A second reason for the importance of truth is that, in general, deception has worse consequences than nondeception and the consequences of people knowing the truth about themselves are better than the consequences of people not knowing the truth about themselves.

Consider the effects of the practice of truth-telling (or veracity). Trust and confidence are important factors in health care. It may be that trust and confidence themselves have a significant therapeutic effect. (In that case, having recourse to deception in order to produce a placebo effect is risky in as much as it endangers the beneficial effect of trust and confidence.) If truthfulness is a recognized practice in health care then it will help to support that trust and confidence. On the other hand, if deceit and withholding of information are generally practised, this will tend to undermine trust and confidence. One of the bad effects of a practice of suppressing bad news is that good news comes under suspicion. Obtaining a small child's cooperation with a procedure by means of deceitful assurances that the child will not feel a thing is likely in the long term to do more harm than good. The job of other nurses on other occasions will be a bit harder because of the patient's suspicion and the difficulty of conveying to the patient what is going to happen.

One kind of undesirable consequence of deception is that relations with people who know more than one does oneself are likely to become difficult and strained.

Another is that, because deception is hard to maintain indefinitely, it tends to be discovered or at least suspected. This has a damaging effect upon trust between persons; and discovered deception can cause the deceived person great disappointment, feelings of betrayal, etc. Conversely, each act of truthful communication contributes to the building up or sustaining (or both) of trust and confidence.

If one person knows things which are importantly relevant to central concerns of another person but are unknown to that person, then the two people are not going to be able to communicate and relate to one another in an open and unstrained way on matters connected to those concerns. And to the extent that one area of communication and mutual understanding is thus excluded their scope for relating to one another is distorted. Maintaining a full human relationship with a person involves candour. It involves not wilfully keeping or placing the other party in a world of facts different from the world of facts one occupies oneself; relating to a person is a matter of continually building and maintaining a common world with that person. (For discussion of the difficulties faced by a wife who has the task of keeping her husband from knowing that he is dying, see Parkes, 1975, pp. 84–85)

Information about a person's health, recovery from injuries, etc. is, in the ordinary way of things, importantly related to central concerns of that person. If there is serious discrepancy between a patient's knowledge of such matters and the information that those caring for the patient have, then communication between them is going to be restricted or distorted.

In section 7.1, we noted reasons for truthfulness supported by the principle of autonomy. The reasons for truthfulness discussed in the present section are reasons supported by the principle of beneficence: an important part of the case for thinking truthfulness important consists in arguing that truthfulness can do good and avoid harm. The considerations in this and the previous section, even if they are found convincing, do not establish that people always ought to be told the truth about themselves. What they do establish, though, is that, where for very good reason people are permitted to remain ignorant of important truths affecting themselves, there is a loss in terms of autonomy and interpersonal relationships. That the loss was worth incurring does not alter the fact that it is a loss.

Where the right course of action involves deception, the deception could be thought of as a moral cost. As with a financial cost, there will be many occasions where one is entirely satisfied with the transaction and has no regrets. But costs are still costs, even when incurred gladly. The fact that £ 5 may be well spent on some occasions is no reason for throwing money away on other occasions. Likewise, the fact that a deception is right on some occasions is no reason to deceive on other occasions.

7.3 PATIENTS' LIFE-PLANS AND THE BIRTHDAY PRESENT PROBLEM

In section 2.3b we reviewed the notions of personal and impersonal value. The points about autonomy and beneficence just noted in sections 7.1 and 7.2 are reasons for supposing that people's knowing the truth about matters concerning themselves is impersonally valuable. Now let us look at the subject from a different angle and think instead about personal value.

One person's considered and chosen style of life may be one in which pleasantness is accorded a higher rating than truth-of-belief. In the event of such a person's being ill in a way that is serious but deniable (supposing that the truth can be sustainably kept from the person – and such a person is likely to have developed ways of cooperating in benign deception), it is likely that suppressing information about their condition will be the most beneficent course relative to their personal values. In that case, insisting that the person come to terms with the truth would be paternalistic, and there would be good reason not to do it. It would be overruling a person's choice of a way of living their life.

Another person's reflectively preferred style of life may be one in which truth-of-belief is assigned a higher rating than pleasantness. In the event of such a person's being ill in a way that is serious but deniable, it is likely that telling them about their condition will be the most beneficent course relative to their personal values. In that case, withholding the truth would be paternalistic, and there would be good reason not to do it. It would be overruling a person's choice of a way of living their life.

When one person has to make decisions for another in matters of importance and seeks to respect the other person's considered preferences about how to live, an obvious course to take is to ask the other person what their preference in the matter is. If I have to order lunch for you, it is very helpful if I can tell you the options and get you to instruct me about which of them you prefer. However, when the question is whether certain information is to be made known to you, this possibility is not available. I cannot set out the options and ask which one you want me to take. If I say 'You are terminally ill; would you prefer not to be told?' then I have already taken away from you the option of not being told. Since I do not have the possibility of setting out the options for you and asking your preference, I have to find some other way of respecting your considered preferences about how to live your life. I am confronted with a variant of the birthday present problem. Typically the problem facing someone wanting to give a birthday present is to find something that will not be expected by the recipient but which will turn out to be just what the recipient wanted. Some people are good at solving that problem; they are sensitive to and take note of how their friends prefer their lives to be and are thus able to extrapolate those life preferences to new situations. People who dependably give their friends presents that surprise and delight have virtues that people who have to decide on informing patients of poor prognoses could usefully have.

What to do about unwelcome truth, in this perspective, is a matter of judging what a person's chosen way of living is. Thus knowing what to do about unwelcome truth is a matter of being able to judge what a person's chosen way of living is. And the virtue of dealing well with matters of truth will include the cognitive capacity of judging well what sort of life people have chosen to live. It will also involve not waiting until the decision about telling has to be made, but acting at earlier stages in ways which will leave one well-placed to make such judgements, being sensitive to signs of what the person's personal values are, and so on.

A complicating factor is this. People can be wrong about their personal values. (Recall the Midas story: gold was not as important to Midas as he at first thought it was.) The limits of a person's imagination may mean that, even if while in good health they reflect carefully on their priorities, they may fail to do justice to how things will look to them when they are not in good health. To that extent, in addition to judging well what sort of life a person has in fact chosen to live, one may have to judge how the person's choices concerning how to live would be modified in the light of their further experience (including now the experience of being ill). This, too, is a matter of judgement. It *may* be, in some cases, that a person who while healthy thought they would always want to know the worst would while ill prefer comfort to truth. But merely assuming that this is always going to be so is cutting corners; it is cutting out the work of judgement.

7.4 REDUCED AUTONOMY

It is important to keep in view the possibility that a given patient is only imperfectly autonomous. One way in which a person's autonomy might be impaired is through lack of information. Another way is for strong and central elements in the person's motivation to enduringly resist coherent integration into the person's self. Where a person's autonomy is impaired solely or mainly by their lacking information that another person has, aiming to foster autonomy commits the other person to disclosing the information. Where an important factor in the imperfection of a person's autonomy is the lack of a coherent integration of central elements in their motivation, fostering autonomy does not straightforwardly involve conveying information; it rather involves seeking to facilitate the person's moving towards a new integration, a new identity.

Earlier we mentioned that if someone wants to know the truth about their own condition, withholding it is extremely hard to justify. That should now be qualified. If the want is well integrated into a unitary self and is endorsed by the person, then denying it is indeed hard to justify. But suppose that, on the contrary, the person has this want but also has a strong need for reassurance and, far from either of these having become the policy of the entire self, the two are simply pulling the person in two directions without the person having – as is often said – made up their mind. A want that, while present, has not become the person's policy does not have the same claim on others. A want that has become the policy of an integrated self has a claim to be respected as expressing a person's autonomy; a want that has not become the policy of an integrated self does not have that claim on us. The principle of autonomy then points to actions that will support the restoration or development of autonomy rather than the respecting of autonomy that is taken to be already present.

Maintaining a high level of patient information and urging patients to be responsible or co-responsible for their own treatment and the management of their own lives may be desirable in general. However, a patient's coming death does present a special kind of case. The information that one's life is likely to end comparatively soon and much sooner than one had hitherto anticipated is not just another piece of information that needs to be taken into account in one's plans. It differs from other information not just in magnitude (in the magnitude of the potential plan changes that it forces) but in the *kind* of significance it has. It can have a shattering effect on the person who is to die or on persons who will be bereaved. The word 'shattering' is here used advisedly. The different elements in a person's response to such information may be impossible to integrate with one another and with the overall developing pattern of the person's life. Thus it is very likely that the person just will not have a coherent response.

Often an appropriate nursing response to a question, where there is room for serious doubt or disagreement about whether disclosing the relevant information is the correct response, is to seek to learn more about the patient. People do not always choose the best way of achieving what they want; they do not always know what they want. A patient who just wants to voice a deep worry and share it with someone may say 'Am I going to live?' as a (not especially well chosen) way of initiating the conversation that they really want to have. Rather than assume that the patient has made the best choice of opening move, it is often better to seek a clearer indication of what is wanted. One way of doing this may be to ask whether the patient is worried.

Sometimes, of course, a person who asks for information really wants to have that information. Health care workers need to bear in mind that it can be very frustrating for someone who wants information to be met instead with counter-questions. The ploy of responding to the request for information with an enquiry about how the patient feels should not be made into an unthinking routine. It may be appropriate when the patient's autonomy is significantly impaired and not when the patient is unequivocal about what he or she wants.

The aim of promoting or restoring autonomy is of course not the only aim of nursing care. It may be that for some patient no significant measure of autonomy is achievable at all. In that case, other aims of nursing become dominant and the relative importance of the patient's being informed about his or her own condition may diminish.

7.5 NEED TRUTH BE A GUIDING CONCERN?

The decision to withhold information from a patient is one that affects everyone who is party to the information and who has dealings with the patient. In particular it affects all in the health care team; it directly concerns their work. Even if team members other than the doctor do not make acknowledged contributions to the deliberative process leading to the decision, the decision is still a team decision in that the doctor makes the decision not just for herself or himself but for the whole team. Other members of the team will have to participate in implementing the decision and will have to live with its consequences. Taking this into account is a matter of elementary courtesy and consideration even if the decision is the doctor's alone.

An agent faced with a decision on disclosing information about a patient to that patient needs to consider certain questions. This is so whether the agent is an individual (e.g. doctor, nurse, relative) or a group. Some central questions are these:

- whether as a matter of objective value it would be best for this patient to be informed of the truth;
- whether, relative to this patient's considered view of how to live, it would be best for the patient to be informed;
- whether the patient actually wants to be told;
- whether the patient *can* be told (because properly grasping the information might require technical knowledge and a conceptual repertoire that the patient lacks – see Hilfiker, 1985, pp. 56–67);
- how the patient ought to be told; and, if staff shortages make it impossible for the patient to be told in that way, whether it would be better for the patient not to be told at all than to be told in the wrong way;
- how the act of telling or not telling the patient will relate to what other agents do (because, if different members of the health care team are saying different things to the patient, this may merely make the patient confused and frightened);
- whether telling or not telling the patient is going to make life difficult for other health care workers, and whether it is going to affect the care the patient receives.

None of these questions on its own is likely to settle the matter. Deliberating about keeping patients informed cannot in general be reduced to answering one simple question. It would be nice to have a simple formula which could be relied upon to produce a decision in most cases. But, while there are some simple moral ideas which we need to keep a grip on (like the ones set out in the first two sections of this chapter), applying them to concrete situations can be complex because of the other factors in those situations.

There are common arguments for not letting truth be a dominant concern shaping the deliberation of a health team (or the deliberation of someone who will decide on behalf of a health team). We now review four such arguments. They are to the effect that the patient should not be told all about his or her case because (1) it is not possible to convey the truth accurately and comprehensibly to patients (they lack the specialized knowledge and training and perhaps intelligence to grasp it), (2) human knowledge is imperfect and even the professionals cannot be absolutely sure what the truth is and what the future will hold, (3) patients do not want bad news and that preference should be respected, and (4) the effect of bad news can actually be to make the patient's condition worse.

The first argument depends on the idea that what is impossible cannot be morally required. Thus, given that conveying the whole truth with total accuracy in a way that the patient will understand is not possible, it cannot be what ought to be done. But this argument is beside the point. A complete and totally accurate account is not what is wanted. What is wanted is an account of the main points and the practical implications. An expert who has his or her share of imagination can generally find a way of making the main points and the practical implications of some technical matter to a lay person. Good motor mechanics can do it. Doctors ought to be able to. Thus the first argument does not successfully give a reason why patients should not be told their diagnosis and prognosis.

We noted in section 7.1 that indeterminacy in a person's plan can mean a lower level of autonomy. We should also note, however, that some indeterminacy is inevitable and that indeterminacy in details and relatively insignificant factors does not reduce autonomy at all. Ignorance of the main practically significant points of what is going to happen to me reduces my autonomy; ignorance of technical details may well not reduce my autonomy at all.

The second argument gives the imperfection of human knowledge as a reason for not telling the patient what the professionals believe to be the case. And it would indeed be wrong of health professionals to misrepresent something as certain or foolproof when it is doubtful or risky. But the elusiveness of absolute certainties is not in general a reason for keeping the information from the patient.

> Not knowing the whole truth should not prevent anyone from being told what is actually known and what can reasonably be conveyed to the person by the informant.
>
> (Schröck, 1980, p. 141)

The third argument will detain us longer. It is that since patients do not want bad news they should not be given it.

> One of the astonishing things about patients is that the more serious the disease, the more silent they are about its portents and manifestations. . . . patients with organic disease are very chary about asking point blank either the nature or the outcome of their ailment. They sense its gravity, and the last thing in the world they wish to know is the truth about it; and to learn it would be the worst thing that could happen to them.
>
> (Collins, 1981, p. 65)

Describing a case where he was taken in by the apparent sincerity of a patient's request to know the truth, Collins describes the result of his complying with that request:

> The light of life began to flicker from the fear that my words engendered, and within two months it sputtered and died out. He was the last person in the world to whom the truth should have been told. Had I lied to him, and then intrigued with his family and friends, he might be alive to-day.
>
> (Collins, 1981, p. 66)

One cannot tell from the text whether the distortion of family relations was a cost that Collins (1981) judged would have been worth paying, or whether it did not enter his calculations. In another case, deception paid rich dividends:

> Months of apprehension had been spared him by the deception, and he had been the better able to do his work, for he was buoyed by the hope that his health was not beyond recovery. Had he been told the truth, black despair would have been thrown over the world in which he moved, and he would have carried on with corresponding ineffectiveness.
>
> (Collins, 1981, p. 66)

An important point about this case is that the deception is presented as worthwhile because it enabled the patient to see to its conclusion a project which was of the greatest importance to him. Collins (1981) wants to convince his readers that patients with serious diseases do not want to know the truth and that learning it would be the worst thing to happen to them; he wants his readers to hold fast to this conviction even when their experience of a particular patient is contrary to it. (Otherwise, they will be taken in by patients' false protestations of wanting the truth.) But in the quoted case of benign deception, the doctor's judgement concerning the individual patient played a crucial role; the doctor judged both that seeing the project through really was the most important thing for the patient and that the patient would not see the project through if he knew the truth. Here the justification for deception depends on the doctor's having considerable knowledge of the individual patient and insight into the patient's personal values.

Thus Collins (1981) does not succeed in giving us good reason to be guided by a general presumption that the seriously ill had better not be told. If anything, his examples point up the need for the health care team to have the kind of knowledge of a patient that can best be obtained in the context of sustained open communication. Keeping patients *generally* well informed enables members of the team to form a well-founded impression as to whether a particular patient prefers knowing all and being in control or prefers to live from day to day while others do the worrying. The day to day practice of offering the patient open communication enables the carers to receive feedback from the patient as to whether information is wanted or not.

The fourth argument, starting from a general presumption that withholding unwelcome news is going to protect people from harm, has equally little to be said for it. The consideration that the truth is sometimes harmful is no justification for a general policy of withholding unwelcome information given that such a policy would be undesirable on other grounds. To be justified in withholding information on the ground that the patient may not be able to cope with it, one would need to have reason to believe that *this particular* patient is one who would not be able to cope with it.

At a more mundane level, the chances of unwelcome diagnoses harming people have to be weighed against the chances of people being harmed by uncertainty in a climate where doctors are known to be reticent about diagnoses of cancer. Knowing that reassuring vagueness can be a sign that you have got cancer, a patient may become suicidal as a result of reassuring vagueness.

Granted that there are some cases in which the truth is better not told, a deliberating agent has to be awake to the possibility that the present case is one of them. However, there is an all-too-human tendency to think that something is the case when one *wants* it to be the case. So, when deliberation is moving towards the conclusion that telling the truth would be out of place, the deliberation needs to include a review of the agent's own motives. ('Am I really thinking about the patient, or am I just dreading the task of telling the patient the worst?')

Having reviewed these arguments, we have not found good reason to change the presumption that truth should be a guiding concern in relations with patients.

7.6 VERACITY AND TEAM OBLIGATIONS

We noted in section 7.3 that sustainable success in solving many cases of the birthday present problem involves knowing the recipient well enough to have a good idea of their conception of how to live. Standard contemporary accounts of the nature and aims of nursing make getting to know the patient an integral part of nursing care. The nursing process involves a preliminary assessment of which forming views as to the patient's chosen style of life is an important part; the process also involves continuing review of the preliminary assessment and alertness to signs that it should be altered. Thus when the process is implemented the nursing members of the team will be particularly well placed to contribute to the health care team's appreciation of the patient's preferences concerning how to live.

Above, we have been discussing considerations that might enter into deliberation concerning whether the truth should be told to a person or withheld. However, we should note that continuing to withhold the information may involve sustaining a deception over a long period, and that this may turn out not to be practically possible or – even if possible – far too much of a strain on those who have to sustain the deception. These points have not been mentioned in the discussion so far because we wished to see whether there might be good reason to tell the truth even where deception is not hard.

One question concerning unfavourable prognoses is whether the patient ought to be told. If they ought to be told then there is an obligation to tell them. But who has that obligation? One often hears or reads of the dilemma of the nurse who is suddenly asked for information by the patient but who does not know how much the patient already knows, or has had no instructions about communicating information to this particular patient or has had instructions not to tell the patient anything. When our attention is focused on this typical case, we tend to suppose that if the patient ought to be told then the obligation to tell the patient falls on the nurse. Yet the nurse who makes unauthorized disclosures to the patient or even goes against explicit instructions may face very unpleasant consequences because of the power relations among different members of the health care team. Demanding that the nurse do that is asking nurses to be heroic in defying the system. It seems unreasonable to say that nurses should have to choose between heroism on the one hand and unethical behaviour on the other. It is a harsh morality that places the full burden of responsibility on the individual nurse when the creation and sustaining of the problem is due to other parties.

We should consider here the possibility that if there is an obligation to tell the patient the obligation falls, in the first instance, not on any individual but on the health care team. In the case where a patient ought to be told something, then, the team's actions should be such that the patient gets told. If a group of people or an institution has an obligation, it does not follow that any individual has exactly that obligation. (A building society may owe me money without it being the case that an individual employee or officer of the building society has an obligation to hand over money to me.) Likewise, if there is an obligation on the health care team to tell the patient something it does not follow that that very same obligation also falls on the individual nurse.

However, even if the individuals belonging to a group do not have exactly the same obligation that the group has, they are likely to have some related obligations. Let us dwell for a moment on the comparison between an individual's deliberation and a group's deliberation. An individual may think her deliberating on some important matter has been done badly (because, for example, she omitted to take some significant factor into account). In that case she has an obligation to go over it again if she has a chance to. A group's deliberation is the process by which a decision concerning the group's conduct is taken. A member of a group may have reason to think that the group's deliberation on an important matter has been done badly (because, for example, certain important information – perhaps about the patient's life preferences or present state of suspicion and anxiety – was not available or did not receive its proper place in the deliberation). In that case, the group member has an obligation to take whatever opportunity there is of getting the deliberation restarted and securing due prominence for the relevant information.

Similarly, an individual member of a group who has reason to think that the group's deliberative procedures are chronically defective has an obligation to take such steps as there is opportunity for towards getting the deliberative procedures changed. It may be that this is a matter of changing hospital policy or long established practice and that there is little scope for a junior nurse to do anything much about it at all. Still, it is important that the nurse retain a sense of the need for change so that she will not have forgotten it by the time she does have a voice that can be heard. The ability to retain a sense of moral unsatisfactoriness even where the unsatisfactory things cannot be changed is a virtue; it is one of the virtues that are relevant to coping with matters of truth-telling in nursing.

Trying to get a decision reconsidered or a group's procedures changed may be a difficult matter. It may need careful thought, thorough preparation, considerable tact and shrewd judgement about how various people might react. The relevant qualities of character are thus part of the bundle of virtues that are relevant to matters of truth-telling.

7.7 DELIBERATION ABOUT TRUTH-TELLING

We have noted (at the end of section 2.2) the wisdom of being alert to facts about oneself that could distort one's deliberation. This can be particularly relevant in situations requiring a decision about giving a patient information about himself. Part of the process of deliberation on what to do is considering whether fears or prejudices or biases of one's own might lead to distortion of one's assessment of the relevant considerations. If I am very fearful of entering into what might be a painful area of discussion with a person, I may tend to over-estimate the force of some of the reasons for keeping off the subject. On the other hand, it might be that, because of a previous occasion when information was wrongly withheld from a patient, my unresolved feelings of guilt obscure my appreciation of the present situation and bias me in favour of disclosure. No doubt it is impossible to be sure of eliminating such distorting factors from one's deliberation. But simply being aware of them can help to reduce distortion.

An appreciation of the situation will take in many factors: what the truth is (which could be conveyed to or withheld from the patient or client), how much the patient knows already, whether the patient's wishes are clear, what scope there is for getting clearer indications of those wishes, what other parties are involved (other members of the health care team, family, friends), whether other parties have deliberated on the same issue and arrived at relevant conclusions, and so on.

A review of possible courses of action will take in the possibilities of telling the patient outright, encouraging the patient to articulate his hopes and fears concerning the information, acknowledging the patient's question and undertaking to raise with others the question of his being fully informed, pretending not to hear and various other evasions. In considering different possibilities, one would have to take into consideration such constraints as limitations of time, the undesirability of starting things one cannot finish, and so on.

Some of the principles of nursing ethics may connect up with factors in the situation to produce reasons for acting one way or another. If the situation is one in which not the patient but a relative of the patient is making an enquiry and giving the information would mean telling the relative more than the patient has yet been told, then the principle of confidentiality may apply to the situation to produce a reason for declining to answer the question. If the situation is one in which the patient is asking about a minor departure from the usual routine and the true answer is that a consultant has made a mistake, a principle of loyalty may come into play to give a reason for withholding the explanation. If the situation is one where the patient is anxiously asking about his condition and there is reason to think that a truthful answer would produce fear, bewilderment, depression or other harm, the principle of nonmaleficence gives reason to withhold the truth. If the situation is one where there is good reason to think that deception will produce good results, either in the context of treatment or in the context of research then the principle of beneficence gives reason for deception.

Thus other principles besides that of veracity could enter into the nurse's deliberation. Such principles relate to reasons for supposing that one action or another is what she ought to do. It may be that she finds other considerations arising as to what she ought to do, other than those underwritten by general principles of nursing ethics. She will also have to take account of considerations of value: considering one course of action or another, she will note what the likely consequences of that course of action would be and what is good and what is bad about those consequences.

In the course of deliberation, persuasive reasons may take shape for a deceptive course of action. In such a case it is worth applying three tests; namely, considering whether there is a nondeceptive alternative (the Nondeceptive Alternative test), asking oneself 'Would I be content for a comparable lie to be told to me in a comparable situation?' (the Golden Rule test), and considering whether the reasons for the deception would satisfy a public of reasonable persons (the Publicity test) (see Bok, 1980, especially Chapter Seven, for further discussion). The mere fact that deception occurs for a good purpose does not suffice to justify it. Actually discussing the reasons with other people is probably the best way of implementing the last of these tests. In matters of ethical deliberation, two heads can be very much better than one.

The mood of our times seems favourable to keeping patients informed. We have tried to suggest here that there is good reason for this and consequently that considerations of veracity deserve a comparatively substantial role in practical ethical deliberation.

7.8 TRUTH AND VIRTUE

It is in some people's character to cope well with practical problems concerning truth. Let us consider what traits of character are relevant.

At its narrowest, honesty is a reluctance to deceive. Some people lie habitually. Some people's habit is swiftly to size up where their advantage lies or what will keep them the centre of attention and then say whatever will secure their advantage or keep them the centre of attention; they do not care whether it is true or not, but care only whether it will have the desired effects. The habits and concerns of an honest person are different. An honest person cares about truth. While perhaps she cares about personal advantage or being the centre of attention, she does not care about these things in such a way as seriously to consider speaking falsely for their sake. What comes naturally to her is to speak the truth. A concern for truth will guide her relations with other people and will be reflected in her habits of thought and communication. Even people who are not honest will attach special weight to information that they have from someone they know to be honest. That information makes the bigger impression on them because they knew that it was not selected for the impression it would make upon them.

To an honest person, it will not be a matter of indifference whether patients are well- or ill-informed as long as they are happy. Where someone else might be inclined to say 'I really can't see that it makes any difference', the honest person, even where satisfied that deception is the right course, will find the difference plain to see and not hazy or obscure. She will have a sense – that develops with experience – of what it is appropriate for people to know about themselves and what it is inappropriate for them not to know. She will be quick to sense that something is wrong when someone does not know something they ought to know – if, for example, moments after signing a consent form, a patient says 'What are they going to do to me?'

An honest person will be distressed by being caught up in someone else's deception and will be deeply uneasy in a set of social or working arrangements of which deception is a regular and firmly established part. That someone is ignorant of something relevant to central concerns of theirs will be a matter of unease to the honest person.

An honest person does not always tell the truth and does not always unhesitatingly supply whatever information another requests. Suppose that someone, on being asked for certain information, first takes into consideration whether the disclosure of the information could harm someone or would be an unwarranted exposure of someone else's personal affairs or would be giving away something which the interlocutor has no business knowing. The person's taking these things into account is not a sign of dishonesty. With experience, an honest person comes to be better at understanding situations, at noting features of situations which relate to such considerations, and thus better able to cope with practical problems concerning truth. Also with experience will grow a sensitivity to what is being asked and a sensitivity to signs of how much another is ready to be told.

An honest person may have reservations about speaking the truth on a particular occasion. But those reservations will not be self-serving ones. Part of the cognitive side of honesty is a sense of the limits of the entitlement to be told the truth. Another part of the ability to cope well with truth-related problems is courage and firmness in refusing to give information, e.g. in saying 'I'm sorry, I can't tell you that'. However, avowedly not answering the question will sometimes tell the other person part of what he or she improperly wants to know. In that case the honest person may have to deceive.

A dishonest person may suppress some information, not for the benefit of the enquirer but for the sake of a quiet life. The dishonest person may like to think of herself or himself as being honest; in that case he or she may achieve a self-deception to the effect that certain information – which she or he prefers to suppress – is really just unwanted technicality, boring and superfluous detail, etc. It is wise to be aware of the possibility that one is thus deceiving oneself. The tests mentioned at the end of 7.7 are aids to avoiding such self-deception.

The deliberation of an honest individual will be guided by a leading concern with truth. She will choose a deceptive course of action where that is clearly the right course. Her reasons for choosing the deceptive course will be other things that she cares about in the way she cares about truth. And, in such cases, she will retain a sense of the moral cost involved in deception.

If a team is to have the virtue of honesty, its deliberations – like those of an honest individual – will be guided by a leading concern with truth. Part of the moral task of team members is to keep alive such a concern in the team, so that it continues to be an understood thing within the team that truth counts for something and that deception is a moral cost. Again, if the team is to have the qualities needed for coping well with truth-related problems, it will need to be able to form team judgements of what people ought to know, what they want to know and what they are ready to know. Here, too, individuals in the care team may need to be alert to ways of developing these abilities in the team as a whole. As noted at the end of section 7.6, this may not be easy. The person who is good at it will have such qualities as patience, tact and sensitivity. Making a dependably good job of problems about truth involves quite a range of qualities of character. It is not reducible to a simple rule. As Chapter Five suggests, it may even involve confronting pervasive inequalities of power within the health care delivery system.

EIGHT

Abortion

Nurses caring for pregnancy termination patients have to face a range of feelings and questions from time to time: for example, how to respond if the patient seems doubtful or guilty about the termination, or what feelings and thoughts are appropriate about a foetus that may be comparable to some of the premature babies that get nursed through to normal infancy. Some of the questions that arise concern the rights or wrongs of abortion and the status of the foetus. We shall look at these questions in the present chapter.

8.1 WHAT IS ABORTION?

When abortion is discussed as a moral problem, most people have in mind the moral legitimacy of intentionally terminating the life of an embryo or foetus either for therapeutic or for other reasons. (For the rest of this chapter we shall for simplicity's sake usually use only the term 'foetus'.)

However, two points ought to be noted. First of all, not all abortions are intentionally brought about or induced; spontaneous abortions also occur and are believed to account for at least 70% of all conceptions. It might be thought that such abortions pose no moral problems as they are natural occurrences – nature's way, perhaps, of disposing of malformed embryos. However, much health care activity is aimed at altering or preventing natural occurrences. Consider how you would respond if, for example, an acquaintance were to say to you 'Cancer is a naturally occurring phenomenon, so we should let it take its course and not attempt to treat it'.

Second, abortion is sometimes described as the intentional termination of a pregnancy. As things stand at present to terminate a pregnancy is, because of the abortifacient techniques employed and the fact that ectogenesis (the growth and development of a foetus in an artificial womb) has not been fully developed, to kill a foetus. But this is not always so. In the case of very late abortions, there have been instances where foetuses have been born alive. If abortion is the intentional termination of a foetus's life then the abortion procedure is not complete until the foetus has been not only removed from the womb but also killed. However, if abortion is merely the intentional termination of a pregnancy, once a pregnancy has been terminated, subsequent killing of the foetus is not a part of the abortion procedure. How abortion is characterized may make a big difference to the moral conclusions that are reached about abortion.

Furthermore, it might seem that, if ectogenesis became a reality and a woman's pregnancy could be ended by transfer of the foetus from a natural to an artificial womb, the moral problems posed by abortion would be transformed. But if ectogenesis is possible, how many women will then opt for natural child bearing and birth? If none do, does that mean that abortion disappears as a moral issue? Only if you believe that the moral problem of abortion is concerned with the intentional termination of a pregnancy; but if you believe the moral issue is concerned with the intentional termination of the life of a foetus then abortion remains as a moral issue. For foetuses in either a natural or an artificial womb can have their lives terminated.

8.2 ARE ANY REASONS FOR ABORTION GOOD ENOUGH?

Suppose that in some piece of deliberation, abortion features as one of the practical options at stage 2. What reason or reasons would be good enough to justify morally a stage 5 decision for abortion under present-day conditions? There are three possibilities to be considered:

1. no reason is good enough
2. some reasons are good enough
3. any reason is good enough

Let us call these the no-reason view, the some-reason view, and the any-reason view. They are views about what, from a moral point of view, should happen at stage 4.

There are various reasons why abortion might be considered. Here are some possible ones:

- the woman is herself virtually a child
- the woman already has more children than she can manage
- having a child at this time will interfere with a career
- having a child at this time will involve loss of earnings

- the woman is a rape victim
- the woman is a sexually-abused eleven-year-old
- the woman has already had three children by Caesarian section
- the woman was deserted by her partner when he learned of the pregnancy
- the woman is severely mentally defective
- the woman is homeless
- the foetus is believed to be defective
- the woman's life or health is seriously threatened.

Each of the considerations listed – and the list could go on – could be a reason for abortion. However, if the no-reason view is correct then, for the purpose of finding out whether abortion is justified in a particular case, the reason or reasons for abortion in that case do not need to be considered. This is because, no matter what the reasons for abortion are in a particular case, they are never going to be strong enough to justify abortion. While considerations like the above might continue to feature in an agent's deliberation, they can properly support only courses of action other than abortion.

Why might no reason be good enough to justify abortion? One line of thought is that, from the moment of conception when the egg is fertilized by the sperm, terminating the foetus's existence is just as wrong as killing any human person. The idea here is that the foetus should have ultimate respect, this being at all times such a powerful reason *against* abortion that no reason *for* abortion can outweigh it.

By contrast, it might be thought that personhood is acquired at birth or later and that, before birth, the foetus is just so much tissue. This line of thought would support the any-reason view. If this view is correct, then not much attention need be given to the particular reasons in an individual case; for, whatever reasons they are, they are bound to be good enough.

The thought underlying the no-reason view is that there is one reason against abortion which is so powerful that, whatever the reasons for abortion in a particular case, they can never outweigh that one supreme reason against. The thought underlying the any-reason view is that there is nothing about foetuses in general that would be a decisive reason for not aborting them, so that any reason at all for abortion in a particular case is a good enough reason.

The some-reason view might seem plausible just because the no-reason view and the any-reason view are found hard to believe. Can a reason against abortion really be so powerful that you can be certain in advance that no reason for abortion will ever be strong enough to rival that reason against? And yet can justifying abortion really be so very easy as the any-reason view would make it? The difficulty of sustaining a 'yes' answer to either question prompts the thought that the some-reason view is correct.

Again, to the extent that the no-reason view and the any-reason view depend, respectively, on decisive importance being attributed to the moment of conception and to the moment of birth, it might be thought that both views are wrong because the changes occurring at those two moments are less important than changes which occur in the interval between them.

A different ground for taking the some-reason view is that a person has a right not to have far-reaching and enduring changes to their life-plans imposed upon them by factors beyond what they can reasonably be regarded as responsible for. Here the suggestion is that non-frivolous reasons for continuing with prior life-plans can be sufficient to justify abortion. We consider this suggestion further in later sections.

The some-reason view might also be taken simply because some reasons for abortion seem so exceptionally powerful as to override other considerations. Two reasons which may be thought to have this status are that the pregnancy has come about as a result of rape and that the foetus is showing signs of abnormal development. These suggested reasons are considered in sections 8.4 and 8.5 below.

8.3 THE ARGUMENTS REFINED: MORALLY SIGNIFICANT DIVIDING LINES

Why might we want to take the no-reason view? An extremely important line of thought is the following:

> Killing an innocent human being is wrong.
> A foetus is an innocent human being from the moment of conception.
> Inducing abortion is killing a foetus.
> So inducing abortion is wrong.

Note that the conclusion here follows logically from the premises. Anyone who accepts the premises but denies the conclusion is contradicting themselves. So to find out whether this argument compels you to take the no-reason view you have to find out whether you accept the premises. And even then you have to consider whether the wrongness of abortion – which is clearly a reason for deciding against abortion in any case – is so powerful a reason that it can never be outweighed in a particular case by reasons for an abortion.

Note that the first premiss is easier to defend than an unqualified principle forbidding the taking of any human life. Accepting the first premiss does not oblige you to say that all killing of humans is wrong. One can believe that certain kinds of killing are right (e.g. the killing of convicted murderers in capital punishment, or combatants in warfare) and still accept the first premiss.

This argument will be considered more fully in section 8.9. For now, let us look at a line of thought that might lead one to take the any-reason view:

Prior to entering the human community at birth, a foetus is of no moral significance.
So inducing abortion infringes no moral restriction on killing.

Here the idea is that any prohibition on killing innocent human beings will start to apply only at birth, so that it does not rule out killing a foetus. Birth can be thought of as especially significant because it is then that the child enters a human community and relationships with its immediate family can begin to develop.

In introducing the principle of autonomy in section 2.4, we made a contrast between things and persons. We then noted that, whereas it may be all right for things to be used merely as means, the autonomy principle rules out using persons merely as means. This may suggest that everything we encounter is to be classified as either a thing or person. We now wish to introduce another term and say that an entity has **moral standing** if, because of what it is, there are moral restrictions on its use as a means. According to the autonomy principle, persons have moral standing. It may be that some beings other than persons have moral standing. And it may be that the moral standing of some beings is a less weighty consideration (to be taken into account at stage 4) than the moral standing of some other beings. From time to time in the discussion that follows we shall make reference to the possibility that human foetuses or embryos have moral standing.

Now consider the argument about moral standing starting at birth. There are reasons to be sceptical about this. First of all, no significant change in the internal development of the foetus occurs at birth; indeed many prematurely born infants are significantly less well developed than foetuses which, having gone to term, are about to be born. Second, even though a child enters into family relationships after birth, it may be that significant bonding occurs before birth, so that birth marks not a change in moral standing but a mere change in location from a uterine to a non-uterine environment. On the other hand, some thinkers consider the notions of community and membership of a community important enough to outweigh these difficulties. They think that persons are *essentially* social beings, so that one's being a person is inseparable from one's being a member of a community or society, rather than being individuals who happen to be in communities but could equally have been quite alone.

Let us explore for a few moments the idea that neither conception nor birth marks a morally significant dividing line. Perhaps some appropriate dividing line can be found between these two. One suggestion is that viability – the time at which the foetus could survive outside the womb – is a morally significant dividing line. This would go some way towards meeting the sense that, because a baby just before birth is very similar to a newborn baby, birth cannot be the decisive boundary. At the same time it would go some way towards meeting the sense that ultimate respect has something to do with membership of a community of distinct human beings. For it suggests that such respect is appropriate when an unborn baby has the capacity to exist as a distinct living being, by contrast with the nonviable foetus whose dependence on its host means that it has to be regarded as part of the woman's body.

However, viability is now thought of as starting 24 weeks after conception and, with new technological advances, it is probably set to start even sooner (ectogenesis would date viability from conception). There may be difficulties about the very idea of a variable dividing line marking off moral standing which is dependent on the development of medical technology, and varying between societies with their various levels of technological development. Further, a foetus of 24 weeks, although technically viable, does require the sophisticated technology of a neonatal intensive care unit for its survival. At that stage, it might seem as dependent as the foetus still in the womb. On the other hand, it is not immediately clear whether the distinction between independent and dependent existence can carry the moral weight required of it. For, if we consider adult persons, moral standing is not necessarily affected by dependence on life support machines.

Other possible dividing lines lying between conception and birth are quickening and implantation. Quickening is the first occasion when the pregnant woman experiences foetal movement. It is difficult to accept that this experience is of any moral significance because it would involve an acceptance of the implausible suggestion that an individual whose movement is unexperienced lacks moral standing. There is a traditional, but now discarded, Catholic doctrine that experienced foetal movement represents the arrival of the soul and the acquisition by the foetus of moral standing (later in the case of a girl foetus than in the case of a boy foetus). It was held that unensouled foetuses could be aborted.

Implantation is the implanting of the foetus in the wall of the womb and occurs between the sixth and the thirteenth day after conception. Without such implantation the foetus would not survive. If membership of the human community is thought of as being reached by stages of first being physically united with and then becoming separated from someone who already is a member, implantation might present itself as an important beginning. It many seem implausible, though, to claim that this physically necessary condition for continuing development confers moral standing on the foetus.

If good reason could be found for taking implantation to be the decisive dividing line, it would support the idea that 'morning after' contraceptive pills and intrauterine contraceptive devices (which prevent foetuses implanting) are morally acceptable, even though there is a case for regarding them as abortifacients. It would also suggest that there is no obligation on us to endeavour to locate and save unimplanted foetuses.

It was noted above that the some-reason view might be attractive just because the dividing lines associated with the no-reason view and the any-reason view can look implausible. However, one may find oneself inclined to the some-reason view not by considerations about dividing lines but rather by the compelling power of some reasons. We now consider two such reasons, namely, rape and foetal abnormality.

8.4 RAPE AS A REASON FOR ABORTION

Michelle is a 19-year-old rape victim who now finds out that she is pregnant. Her ordeal has left her tense, anxious, and prone to nightmares. Previously a cheerful, friendly young woman, she is not now expected to recover her happy disposition in the foreseeable future. The prospect of carrying and giving birth to the child of the man who raped her fills her with revulsion.

Michelle has given little thought to abortion in the past. She has never been a convinced advocate of abortion. As she never expected the issue to touch her personally, she had not got round to considering what she thought about it beyond feeling sorry and sympathetic towards the two or three people in her acquaintance who had had abortions.

Now she has very mixed feelings. First, she wishes the whole thing had never happened and would be intensely relieved if she were to wake up and find that it had all been a dreadful dream. She would be likewise relieved, as far as the pregnancy is concerned, if she were to have a spontaneous early miscarriage or if it were to turn out that there had been a mistake and she was not pregnant after all. She does not regard the new life within her as anything of hers; for her it is rather something of the man's that is still being forced upon her. At the same time, having always regarded abortion as in some way regrettable, she is not content simply to choose it now as one of her options. In addition to her other troubles, she resents being placed in a position where she must choose between having an abortion and continuing with this pregnancy.

If rape is a good enough reason for abortion then those caring for Michelle may have the task of helping her to bring together her different thoughts and feelings on the matter and integrate them into a coherent attitude of being wholeheartedly for having abortion or wholeheartedly against it (to make up her mind, as we say). This caring task would be set by the nursing aim of promoting and/or restoring autonomy. Alternatively, the caring team may act paternalistically in view of Michelle's reduced autonomy and, having first decided that it is in Michelle's best interest for the pregnancy to be terminated, ease Michelle towards an acceptance of the conclusion that she should have an abortion.

If no reason – not even any of the reasons arising from the fact that a pregnancy has come about by rape – is a good enough reason for abortion then helping Michelle towards a decision without prejudice to either the abortion option or the continued pregnancy option is not an appropriate goal of nursing care. In this case, Michelle's coming to the conclusion that what she wants, all things considered, is an abortion is to be regarded with sympathy and understanding but not to be endorsed; her making up her mind for an abortion is itself a problem and not a step towards a solution of her problem.

A central argument for the no-reason view involves the idea that a foetus is a human being essentially like any other human being (see section 8.3, above). Suppose the ill-effects of a rape could be alleviated by killing some innocent third party. You may think that, all the same, the innocent third party should not be killed. According to that argument for the no-reason view, this is exactly Michelle's situation. Although there are powerful reasons in favour of Michelle's having an abortion if that is what she finally wants, they fail to outweigh the master reason against abortion. Being killed is a worse fate than being pregnant through rape. So Michelle's plight counts for less than the plight of the foetus.

The reasons for abortion in a case such as Michelle's are considerable. Nevertheless, it is hard to see how they could be sufficient to justify the killing of an innocent third party. It therefore looks as though, if rape is to be a good enough reason to justify abortion, the life of a foetus has to be regarded as counting for less than the lives of other human beings. And if the life of a foetus does indeed count for less than the lives of other human beings then it cannot be ruled out that there will be other reasons – apart from those relating to rape – which will also be sufficiently powerful to justify abortion.

8.5 FOETAL ABNORMALITY

John and Fiona had been trying for years to have a child. Fiona, now in her early forties, had practically given up all hope of ever conceiving. However, the unexpected happened and she found herself pregnant.

On attending the antenatal clinic she was advised that she ought to have an amniocentesis test as, given her age, there was a significant possibility of the child's being handicapped and, in particular, having Down's Syndrome. It was also pointed out that it was the policy of the centre to which she would be referred not to give this test, in view of the cost and possible risks to the foetus, unless she would agree in advance to have an abortion if the test showed evidence of foetal abnormality.

Fiona was shattered. This was a baby she wanted desperately, and she was horrified to hear that it might be handicapped. To be told, moreover, that the test which might set her mind at rest would be conducted only if she agreed to have an abortion should the test show signs of abnormality was almost too much for her to cope with.

She discussed the situation with John. Both felt they would find it difficult to cope with a handicapped child, but at the same time this was the child they had waited for for so many years. Fiona reflected on the issue. Why should a foetus which shows signs of abnormality be aborted when children suffering from the same disability are not killed? If it is wrong to kill such a child or indeed adult, why should it be acceptable to abort the foetus? She had always believed abortion was wrong, partly for personal reasons in that she could not accept foetuses being killed when she so desperately wanted to be pregnant, and partly because she felt abortion was simply murder. But if she was being offered the possibility of an abortion it was quite clear that foetal life was not been given the same status as postfoetal life.

In the end, Fiona and John felt that the risk of having a handicapped child was too great and their ability to cope too doubtful. So she had the test. Fortunately, no evidence of abnormality was found, and Fiona and John are now the proud parents of a healthy girl.

Sally and Frank Wilson are a married couple in their twenties with no children so far. Two weeks ago Sally had a mild attack of rubella (having somehow missed immunization while she was at school). Now they find that she is in the seventh week of pregnancy. They are eager to have a child but are very distressed at the possibility of their child's being deformed. Their family doctor has already mentioned to them that, under English law, abortion is an option.

In talking the matter over with her friends Jean and Alice, Sally notes that the significant chance of her baby's being seriously handicapped looks like a reason for having an abortion. But Jean and Sally both find themselves wondering whether it is a powerful enough reason (or even really a reason at all).

In many of the cases where there is a significant chance of a foetus developing into a handicapped child, the foetus is in fact developing normally and will (if pregnancy continues) develop into a normal child. But if the *chance* of handicap is a good enough reason for abortion, it would be a good enough reason for terminating many pregnancies where the foetus is in fact developing normally. Jean suspects that it is not a good enough reason in those cases. So she finds herself coming to the conclusion that it is not a good enough reason in any case. As Jean puts it, 'If you make a practice of deciding on abortion whenever there is a significant chance of serious handicap, you are bound to be aborting some foetuses that would have become normal babies. So it's better not to adopt that practice.'

Alice suggests that, if you want to be sure of stopping only the ones that are in fact going to be handicapped, the best thing to do is wait until the baby is born and then, if it is handicapped, let it die. They are all startled by this blunt logic. Then Sally says 'Well, you do have a point; killing defective babies after birth would be pretty bad, but maybe choosing abortion on the strength of a *chance* of a defect is even worse. I am pretty sure I couldn't go along with my handicapped baby's being left to die at birth, so perhaps I shouldn't regard the chance of handicap as a reason for abortion.'

Physical and mental handicaps in human beings often come about as a result of abnormal development of foetuses. In view of this, the likelihood that a particular foetus has such an abnormality may be offered as a reason for abortion. Presumably the reason is more powerful as the likelihood is greater, and as the level of handicap is greater. It may be suggested that a pregnant woman's contracting rubella, with the accompanying risk of deformity in the child, is a sufficiently powerful reason to justify abortion.

However, reflection on the two cases described above prompts two important questions:

1. Is bringing about the abortion of an abnormal foetus morally preferable to waiting until it is born as a defective infant and then killing it?
2. Is aborting many foetuses which might be defective, a significant proportion of them being in fact entirely normal, morally preferable to killing just the defective ones after birth?

If the answer to question 1 is yes, one way of explaining the moral preferability would be to conclude that foetal life does not have the moral standing of postfoetal life. If the answer to question 2 is yes, one way of explaining the moral preferability is to conclude that the moral standing of normal foetuses is less than that of handicapped infants.

Perhaps the two questions are to be answered a different way. Or perhaps some other explanation for affirmative answers is to be found. But acceptance of handicap or the chance of handicap as a sufficient reason for abortion certainly suggests that foetuses are not being accorded the same moral standing as children. This in turn suggests that, if handicap or the chance of handicap is a good enough reason for abortion then there may be other reasons which are also good enough. We thus arrive at a conclusion which echoes that of section 8.4; if the life of a foetus does indeed count for less than the lives of other human beings then it cannot be ruled out that there will be other reasons – apart from those relating to handicap – which will also be sufficiently powerful to justify abortion.

8.6 PREGNANCY AND RIGHTS

Mary is a nineteen-year-old student who has had a number of relationships in her short life and has discovered that she is pregnant. She is determined to have an abortion and confides in her friend Joan.

Joan: Oh you are not. I mean how could you?

Mary: How could I not? Look, this is my life, my body, and I shall do with it what I like.

Joan: You realize, of course, there's no such thing as abortion on demand or as of right in this country.

Mary: I'll do my best to present my case on grounds which are accept-able. But I think it is totally ridiculous that abortion is not avail-able to any woman on any grounds. Whatever way you look at it, it ought to be a *right* for a woman to have an abortion. She is the one within whom the foetus is developing, the foetus is totally dependent on her, and it is her life-plans which will be affected.

Joan: But what about the foetus? Does it not have rights too? You can't just go round killing people because you believe it to be in your interest.

Mary: Look, I know some people do talk about the foetus as a person, but it seems to me that in this case, even if it is a person, my right to an abortion and my rights as a person far outweigh the rights of the foetus. After all, if you state that the foetus is a person, you are only claiming this to prevent me having an abor-tion. And that is totally unacceptable.

In the past few sections we have been focusing on questions concerning the status of the foetus. These questions relate to the value of outcomes. They relate, for example, to the assessment of how bad a motor accident involving loss of life is when the only life lost is that of a foetus. Stage 4 of deliberation frequently and rightly features considerations about how bad or good a certain outcome would be. However, we need to beware of neglecting considerations of other kinds. Often people discussing abortion speak not only about the value of outcomes but also of rights. They may speak of the unborn child having a right to life. They may speak of a person's – including a pregnant woman's – having 'a right to decide what shall happen in and to her body' (Thomson, 1977, p. 133). We were perhaps too hasty in section 8.4 when we said that, despite the substantial reasons for abortion in a case such as Michelle's, it was hard to see how they could be sufficient to justify the killing of an innocent third party. At that stage we were only thinking in terms of the value of outcomes. We were asking how bad it is that Michelle should continue to be pregnant with the rapist's baby and how bad it would be for the foetus's life to be lost. If rights come into these matters then we should consider them as well as the value of outcomes.

Let us recall what the notion of a right involves. If rights are to be taken seriously at all, they have to be understood as setting constraints on the pursuit or production of value. As we noted in Chapter Two, when one talks of individuals having rights one means that their interests or preferences may not be overriden even to achieve great value (see section 2.3d, above).

J. J. Thomson has argued that is it possible to defend abortion on moral grounds even if it is conceded that the foetus is a person and has a right to life. Thomson (1977, p. 133) maintains that a central consideration is the right of the woman 'to decide what shall happen in and to her body'. For convenience, let us speak of this as the woman's right to control her body.

Mary's remarks in the above dialogue show that she has not disentangled considerations about rights from considerations about the status of the foetus and the value of outcomes. In trying to disentangle these considerations, we shall follow Thomson 1977 in considering first of all life-threatening pregnancies and secondly pregnancies which are not life-threatening.

8.7 LIFE-THREATENING PREGNANCIES

It is commonly accepted that the morality of abortion hinges on the status of the foetus. What Thomson 1977 seeks to show is that, even if the foetus has exactly the same moral status as any person, there may still be a moral defence of abortion. This would mean that considerations other than the status of the foetus need to be taken into account in deliberation about abortion.

For the purposes of this discussion, Thomson 1977 concedes that the foetus has full moral standing. Thus it has a full right to life. Equally, of course, the pregnant woman also has a right to life. In addition she has the right to control her body. No doubt the foetus also has the right to control its body.

Now, when we turn to the case of a pregnancy which threatens the life of the pregnant woman (fortunately such cases are rare and getting rarer), Thomas 1977 argues that abortion is justified because, although both parties involved (the woman and the foetus) have a right to life, the pregnant woman has a right to determine what happens to her body. And if her life is threatened by the pregnancy, she has a right to protect her life even if it means the death of the foetus. At bottom, this is an argument from self-defence. In a case of self-defence, a person is justified in taking someone else's life, provided that it is the only means of saving their own life. The abortion case differs from normal self-defence in that the individual killed is innocent; i.e. is not intentionally aiming to kill. (For discussion of self-defence against an innocent threat, see English, 1987 pp. 33–35). But provided that one can justify the taking of innocent lives in self-defence, it is not difficult to justify the taking of life here. Note that the right of self-defence derives solely from the right to life.

So far Thomson 1977 has been considering the rights of the pregnant woman when her pregnancy threatens her life and what she is entitled to do about it. But she also wants to consider how a third party (normally a doctor) ought to react in such situations. One response might be that a doctor can do nothing because both parties involved have a right to life and it would be wrong of the doctor to take sides. Here, Thomson 1977 argues, the right to control one's own body comes into play. Granted that both parties need the use of this body, the fact that it is the woman's body and not the foetus's gives her a special claim to it.

In like fashion, people are not ordinarily forced to donate organs so that close relatives may benefit from an organ transplant. Not agreeing to such a transplant may effectively prevent a life being saved, but compulsion would infringe a person's right to their own organs (even if greater good could be produced by taking them).

8.8 NON-LIFE-THREATENING PREGNANCIES

Carol had been to a party after passing an important examination and met Hugh, a young man she had admired for some time. He suggested they should spend the night together and she agreed. Neither took any precautions against the possibility of Carol conceiving, though Carol did consider the risk, thought it was minimal, and anyway nothing was going to be allowed to spoil her evening. Subsequently Carol was aghast to discover that she was pregnant. Would an abortion, if available, be a morally defensible option for her . . . ?

When Thomson 1977 turns to consider the right of the woman to abort in situations where the pregnancy does not pose a threat to her life, she argues that it is most important to have a clear idea as to what is meant when it is said that the foetus or any person has a right to life. A right to life, she argues, is not a right to be given the means of survival and does not entail a right to the use of someone else's body (Thomson, 1977, p. 119). Depriving a foetus of the continued support of the mother's body would not infringe a right unless the foetus had acquired the right to the use of the mother's body. This account clearly implies that in the absence of such a right abortion is not an injustice. Is this to say, then, that a foetus never has a right not to be aborted? Thomson's 1977 answer (1977, p. 120) is that such a right can be acquired through the woman's actions.

> Suppose a woman voluntarily indulges in intercourse, knowing of the chance it will issue in pregnancy, and then she does become pregnant; is she not in part responsible for the presence, in fact the very existence, of the unborn person inside her? No doubt she did not invite it in. But doesn't her partial responsibility for its being there itself give it a right to the use of her body?

If the foetus has the right to use the woman's body because she is responsible for its being there, to abort the foetus would be to infringe that right. Moreover, in as much as the woman has become responsible for supporting the foetus's life, it would be to violate its right to life.

So, supposing that the foetus has full moral standing, Carol must ask herself whether her actions were such as to give the foetus a right to the use of her body.

Furthermore, as Thomson 1977 points out, 'it might be asked whether or not she can kill it even to save her own life: if she voluntarily called it into existence, how can she now kill it, even in self-defence?' (1977, p. 121). In view of this a self-defence justification of abortion is not so readily available as her earlier argument suggested.

So foetuses conceived willingly have a right to the use of the woman's body and ought not to be aborted because their right to life would be infringed, but foetuses conceived unwillingly through rape or contraceptive failure do not have a right to the use of the woman's body and, if they are aborted, their right to life is not infringed. Thus, by stressing considerations of rights, Thomson 1977 is embracing a some-reason view of abortion.

However, as well as obligations arising from rights, Thomson 1977 acknowledges obligations that are not based on rights. If the cost of inconvenience of greatly helping the very needy is small, one ought to help and display what she calls 'Minimally Decent Samaritanism' (Thomson, 1977, p. 127) even if the beneficiaries of our action do not have a right against us. Within the context of abortion this means that even though a foetus may have no right to the use of a woman's body, it would show a lack of moral decency for the woman not to act in a charitable fashion provided no great sacrifice is demanded. One might even say she ought to do so provided the 'ought' is not believed to derive from a right, because there are no rights here but merely moral decency and the lack of it.

. . . suppose pregnancy lasted only an hour, and constituted no threat to life or health. And suppose that a woman becomes pregnant as a result of rape. . . . Admittedly she did nothing at all which would give the unborn person a right to the use of her body. All the same it might well be said . . . that she *ought* to allow it to remain for that hour – that it would be indecent of her to refuse.

(Thomson, 1977, p. 122)

Thus abortion is *morally permissible* if two conditions which are individually necessary and jointly sufficient are satisfied. The conditions are that the foetus

1. does not have a right to the use of the woman's body, and
2. cannot be sustained without great inconvenience.

Abortion is *morally impermissible* on either of two grounds,

1. the foetus has a right to use the woman's body
2. little effort would be required to continue with the pregnancy.

On this account, Carol has to ask herself not only whether the foetus has a right to the use of her body but also whether the inconvenience or cost to her of continuing the pregnancy is so great that she can decently decline it. Even if different people have different views about what is a small sacrifice and what is a great one, Carol has to make up her mind.

In thinking critically about the Thomson 1977 contribution to the continuing debate on abortion, it is appropriate to enquire how far rights are dependent on specifically assumed responsibilities, whether only those foetuses for which we have taken specific responsibility have a right not to be killed by us, and whether the sharp distinction between what rights demand and what decency requires can be sustained.

To see the difficulty of sustaining it, consider the following. A pregnant rape victim is certainly within her rights in deciding to have an abortion. But if pregnancy only lasted an hour even a rape victim, as we were told, ought as a matter of decency not to have an abortion. But why stop at one hour? What is a small sacrifice anyway? Thomson 1977 gives another example where what decency requires is two months' continuation of pregnancy (Thomson, 1977, p. 127). Why not nine months? For some adherents of the no-reason view, that would not seem a large sacrifice to make. Thus they would be able to achieve with Thomson's 1977 decency considerations exactly what they sought to achieve on the basis of the unborn child's overriding right to life.

More fundamentally, why should considerations of decency be morally influential at all? The answer to this is the value Thomson 1977 accords the foetus. It is because it is foetuses which are aborted, and not stones, that decency matters morally and Thomson 1977 can state that 'while I am arguing for the permissibility of abortion in some cases, I am not arguing for the right to secure the death of the unborn child.' (Thomson, 1977, p. 127.)

Thomson 1977 can accept killing more developed foetuses in abortion only if, given the level of development of the foetus and the abortifacient techniques employed, the death of the foetus is inevitable. If terminating the pregnancy could be achieved without the death of the foetus, say by transferring the foetus to an artificial womb, this would be morally more acceptable. The right to an abortion, on her view, is best thought of as the right to terminate a pregnancy and not the right to secure the death of the foetus.

It is plain that any satisfactory treatment of the abortion issue has to face the question of the moral status accorded to the foetus. In pursuance of that we now turn to examine the foundations of the no-reason view.

8.9 THE NO-REASON VIEW

In section 8.3, we noted the following argument for the no-reason view:

Killing an innocent human being is wrong.
A foetus is an innocent human being from the moment of conception.
Inducing abortion is killing a foetus.
So inducing abortion is wrong.

(See Singer, 1979, for discussion of versions of the arguments considered in sections 8.9 and 8.10.) The first premiss, that killing an innocent human being is wrong, may be taken as expressing a moral rule, corresponding to the idea that each human being has a right to life. By way of exploring this argument, let us ask why the taking of innocent human life is morally wrong.

One suggestion is that *humanness* is special in a way that makes the taking of innocent human life wrong. This amounts to the idea that membership of the species *Homo sapiens* brings with it special rights. A line of criticism that is sometimes directed against this suggestion is that the suggestion embodies a *speciesism* which is as objectionable from a moral point of view as racism or sexism. It may be argued that, just as it is morally unacceptable to treat skin colour or race or sex as a reason for treating some individuals more favourably than others, so it is morally unacceptable to treat species membership as a reason for treating some individuals more favourably than others (see Singer, 1979, pp. 48–54). If this is correct then we have not yet identified exactly why killing innocent human beings is wrong.

A further idea may be introduced at this point, namely the idea that discrimination between humans and non-humans is not arbitrary discrimination because human beings really are special. It may be suggested that there are certain characteristic features of human lives which make this kind of life especially valuable. The distinctively human features of human lives are usually identified as features such as self-awareness, rationality, the capacity to communicate, and the ability to have desires and plans for the future (see, for example, Warren, 1987, p. 16). Thus the idea is that killing human beings is wrong because human beings are rational, self-aware, autonomous persons. (See section 2.4, where we sketched the thinking underlying the principle of autonomy or respect for persons.)

At this point we come to a difficulty. Not all human beings have the features which are suggested as the ground for the preciousness of human life, and the possibility may be admitted that some nonhuman creature may have those features (for perhaps it will turn out that there is intelligent life elsewhere in the universe or that the mental capacities of dolphins or some other creatures are closer to our own than we knew). There are several different lines of thought that may be explored in response to this difficulty. One possibility is this: instead of saying that humans have special rights and they have these rights because of certain psychological features, we might miss out the reference to humans and simply say that beings with those psychological features have special rights. Another possibility to explore is that the members of any species are most appropriately treated in a way that is called for by the characteristics of typical members of that species. Yet another possibility is that individuals are sometimes to be treated not according to what they actually are but according to what they are potentially.

Let us consider first the possibility of simply saying that beings with the appropriate features have the right to life whether or not they are human, and beings which lack those features do not. This would mean that, where taking human life is wrong, its wrongness is due to certain valuable characteristic features. These features are normally, but not always, present within human life; such features may also be present in non-human lives (animal and extraterrestrial) and if they are it is also wrong to take those lives. This account is species-neutral.

Let us see the implications of this for the argument set out above. For convenience, let us use the word 'person' to refer to any being which has the features in question. Then we need to recast the argument by replacing the term 'human being' with the term 'person'. Thus recast, the argument is as follows:

Killing an innocent person is wrong.
A foetus is an innocent person from the moment of conception.
Inducing abortion is killing a foetus.

So inducing abortion is wrong.

The first premiss is normally uncontroversial (although it may be disputed with regard to life-threatening situations – see section 8.7, above). Ordinarily, under present conditions the third is true. However, the second premiss may be thought to present some difficulties. As we are using the term 'person', a person is a being with self-awareness, rationality, etc. Plainly a foetus is not such a being. So the second premiss is false. Thus this version of the argument fails to support the conclusion that abortion is wrong.

The second possibility mentioned above is that the members of any species are most appropriately treated in a way that is called for by the characteristics of typical members of that species. In the present context the issues about foetuses that this raises are best considered with reference to our third possibility, since foetuses are potentially rather than actually members of the species.

8.10 THE POTENTIALITY PRINCIPLE

This brings us to the possibility that individuals are sometimes to be treated not according to what they actually are but according to what they are potentially. Let us modify the argument in line with this idea. We replace the term 'innocent human being' with the term 'potential person'.

Killing a potential person is wrong.
A foetus is a potential person from the moment of conception.
Inducing abortion is killing a foetus.
So inducing abortion is wrong.

As before, we need not be troubled about the third premiss. The second premiss looks unproblematic. However, the first premiss appears to be in need of supporting argument. Here the idea is that, other things being equal, the foetus will develop into an individual having a right to life in virtue of possessing self-awareness, rationality, etc.

As a matter of fact it is true that foetuses do have this potential. But does this count morally? Do potential individuals have the same moral rights as actual individuals? If they do, the justifiability of contraception comes into question; for this practice surely prevents potential people coming into existence. Now it may be thought that this point is irrelevant as what is important about foetuses is that they actually exist and are not merely potential individuals (in the sense in which, for example, unfertilized eggs are). But this is a mistake. The key idea of the potentiality argument concerns not what the foetus actually is but what it potentially is; the key idea is that it is potentially a person. The person which the foetus potentially is is not actual. It is thus comparable to the person that a not-yet-united egg and sperm potentially are. As Glover (1977, p. 122) says, 'If it is cake you are interested in, it is equally a pity if the ingredients were thrown away before being mixed or afterwards.'

As far as the value of foetal life is concerned, what is distinctive about the potentiality argument is the derivative character of the value it accords to the present individual. For the value that it accords to the present foetus is derivative from the value that the future person will uncontroversially have. The present foetus does not have the same properties as the future person will have; so it is by no means obvious that the value of the present foetus is the same as that of the future person.

Considerations about the interests and, perhaps, rights of people in future generations (that is to say, potential people) suggest that there really can be obligations regarding people who are not yet even conceived. So we should not too hastily dismiss the whole idea of a potentiality argument. However, for an argument like the one under consideration here to succeed it would have to be shown that the person's having value at the later time when she or he exists entails the actual foetus's having value at the present earlier time; and it would also have to be shown that, in being derived from the not-yet-actual value of the future person, the value that the foetus has is not too much attenuated.

8.11 ABORTION AND THE CONTEMPORARY SCENE

Writers surveying contemporary attitudes to abortion, adoption and recent advances in reproductive technology often comment on how confused these attitudes seem to be. Abortion may be approved of, but so is adoption which is now very difficult because amongst other things present abortion practices have reduced the number of 'normal' babies to adopt. (There are still quite a number of handicapped babies who could be adopted, but these are much harder to find homes for.) Furthermore, society is willing to spend scarce resources on developing new reproductive technologies to enable couples with infertility problems to conceive and have children of their own while a vastly greater number of foetuses are aborted. On the one hand foetuses are killed, while on the other hand resources are spent enabling women to conceive and still the demand is not satisfied. This seems irrational and contradictory. It is irrational because foetuses are killed while vast sums are spent on generating others. It is contradictory because at one and the same time foetal life is both valued and not valued.

Given the present situation, it is sometimes suggested that the best way forward would be to prohibit abortion and thus make available sufficient babies for adoption; the resources now used to support advances in reproductive technology could then either be saved or spent elsewhere. Furthermore you would have a consistent valuation of foetal life.

Now one fundamental objection to this approach is the restriction it would place on the right of a woman to control her body. Moreover it would deny to the presently infertile woman those future advances in reproductive technology which might alleviate her plight.

However, a more sophisticated statement of the approach just mentioned can be presented. Recall the distinction, made in section 8.1 above, between abortion as terminating a pregnancy and abortion as ending a foetus's life. Let us now take abortion to be simply the intentional termination of a pregnancy. If it were possible to develop an artificial womb (which recent advances in reproductive technology have made more likely) then abortion could take the form of transferring a foetus from a natural to an artificial womb. This would accommodate all the considerations of moral standing and rights mentioned in the foregoing discussion. Foetuses would be saved and would be available for adoption without infringement of the right of the woman to control her own body. It sounds neat, but are there objections to this approach?

8.12 ABORTION AND THE FLIGHT FROM PARENTHOOD

Carol Gilligan (1982) outlines the case of Sandra, a Catholic nurse who decides to have an induced abortion. Sandra sees the options before her as being abortion (which she regards as murder), adoption, and keeping the child. She rules out the third option:

> 'Keeping the child for lots and lots of reasons was just sort of impractical and out'.
>
> (Gilligan, 1982, p. 85)

Sandra has been pregnant before and took the course of adoption on that occasion. Gilligan (1982, p. 85) quotes her as saying

> 'psychologically there was no way that I could hack another adoption. It took me about four-and-a-half years to get my head on straight. There was just no way I was going to go through it again'.

A philosopher, Steven Ross, has argued that, for many women, to seek an abortion is to seek the death of the foetus. For such women, abortion is the intentional termination of the life of the foetus; merely terminating the pregnancy, transferring the foetus to another location to be brought up in the future by another woman or set of parents, is not sufficient. What the woman wants is not simply that the child be somewhere else but rather that that child not exist at all (Ross, 1982, p. 238).

We might be tempted to regard this wish as simply monstrous and not take it seriously as part of a reasonable person's motivation. However Ross (1982) argues that the wish may be linked with considerations about parenthood that we cannot easily dismiss or distance ourselves from. Ross (1982) distinguishes between two concepts of parenthood. On the one hand, we have biological or genetic parenthood where the male and female provide the sperm and the egg to establish the pregnancy. On the other hand, we have social parenthood where the parents are the individuals who look after, sustain and nourish the child. The social parents are commonly also the genetic parents. Adoptive parents furnish a notable example of social parenthood without genetic parenthood. For Ross (1982, p. 240)

> it is usually important to us that the children we raise are the children we have had, and conversely – the more central concern in this discussion – that the children we bear are in fact raised by us. Undoubtedly, this desire is in part instinctual. But it would be a mistake to say it is entirely so; there are reasons for it. In part, it stems from the deep identification parents undoubtedly develop with their children by virtue of the genetic carryover. But it also stems from the more subtle understanding that to raise a child is to influence him or her considerably in a particularly personal way, and that those who *are* so genetically tied to the child have the most legitimate claim to exercise this kind of influence. Thus one anticipates a certain and very special kind of involvement over time that will have this character at least in part because of the initial biological link.
>
> One can of course have good reasons to bear one's child but waive this claim, handing the business of raising it over to another. But we can also have good reasons for avoiding this kind of choice and preventing its attendant difficulties from ever arising. One can, that is, simply want there to be no child at all.

Not all parents feel this way; there are people who freely and quite willingly give their babies up for adoption, participate in surrogacy agreements and who donate eggs or sperm for IVF programmes (for a similar point, see Overall, 1985, pp. 286–287). However, Ross acknowledges this, noting only that many parents do feel in the way he articulates. The issues raised here are undoubtedly difficult and we shall avoid a discussion of them at this stage because we shall be examining them in more detail in the next chapter.

Ross's 1982 general point is that, for many parents in seeking and desiring an abortion, the termination of a pregnancy is not what they have in mind; what they desire is the termination of the life of the foetus. This is what abortion must mean. Subsequent adoption of an unwanted foetus is no answer. Certainly those who encourage and support research to enable infertile women and men to acquire their own biological children cannot ignore Ross's (1982) statements about the importance of biological parenthood; they may, however, wish to dispute the implications of this for the abortion issue.

If Ross's arguments are accepted the 'abortion issue' cannot be transformed simply by redescribing abortion as the termination of a pregnancy resulting in the transfer of a foetus from one location to another, subsequent adoption then following. For Ross 1982, abortion may be concerned with the intentional termination of the life of a foetus and this is not a purely contingent matter reflecting a lack of technological advance but is what, for many women, abortion is about.

What this suggests is that, as long as there continue to be unintended pregnancies, the problem of abortion will continue to be with us. Technological progress may make it possible for the foetus to survive abortion. But this may not spare us the necessity of facing the question whether it may be right to kill foetuses or to fail to save their lives.

NINE

Reproductive technology and allied issues

9.1 INTRODUCTION

Conception used to be closely linked to sexual intercourse. Conception did not occur without sexual intercourse; and one could not count on being able to have sexual intercourse without conception. One of the most significant changes in recent years is the acquired facility to control reproduction. Couples can now plan the number of children they would like to have and, if they so wish, determine to remain childless. In other words, with modern contraceptive methods it is possible to have sexual relations without the risk of conceiving a child. But now we are faced with a new twist to the revolution. With recent developments, the plight of some infertile couples can now be alleviated. Where childlessness occurs not by choice, it is now possible using new technology to enable a woman to become pregnant and give birth to a child which may be genetically the child of one, both, or neither of the partners. In other words, with modern technology ordinary sexual relations are no longer fundamental for the establishment of a pregnancy. With contraception, sexual relations are no longer *sufficient* for the conception of a child (although the sufficiency was always tempered by infertility and the fact that not every copulation results in a procreation); with the new technology, sexual relations are no longer *necessary* for the conception of a child.

But what is this new technology which can be of such benefit to infertile couples? We shall now examine it in some detail and look at a few of the fundamental moral issues it raises.

9.2 ARTIFICIAL INSEMINATION

Artificial insemination occurs when male semen is artificially inserted into a woman's vagina or womb. Two kinds of case have to be considered:

1. In one kind of case, the male partner is physically handicapped or partly infertile. Artificial insemination may then enhance the chances of conception. Artificial insemination with semen supplied by the male partner is known as AIH (artificial insemination by husband). If a child is subsequently born, it is the genetic child of both parents.

2. Cases of another kind are the case where the male partner is completely infertile and the case where there is a risk of transmitting a serious hereditary disease to the genetic child of the male partner. In such cases the semen used would be supplied not by the male partner but by an anonymous donor. In this case we speak of AID (artificial insemination by donor). If a child is subsequently born, it is the genetic child of the mother but not of her partner.

To take an example, suppose Mary and Victor are a married couple in their late twenties who have been trying for a child without success for six years. They are now seriously considering AID as one of the options before them. Two considerations which occur to them might be taken to be reasons for quickly excluding that option. One is the artificiality of AID, and another is the fact that the semen of another man will be used. However, something's being unnatural in the sense of being artificial does not entail any conclusion as to its moral acceptability. (See section 8.1 above, where we noted that something's being natural does not entail that we are obliged to endorse it.) As for the latter consideration it might be thought that the marriage relationship ought to be an exclusive one involving only the two partners, and that the use of a donor's semen is uncomfortably close to adultery. It may be that other factors take away the force of this as a reason for rejecting the AID option. The resemblance to adultery is minimized by donor anonymity, the fact that normal sexual copulation does not take place, and the desire of both partners for AID as a means of overcoming the problem and enabling them to have a child which is genetically related to one of them.

Mary and Victor wonder whether all semen donors should be anonymous. A reason to think this preferable is that it may be difficult to obtain such donations otherwise. A reason for thinking it not preferable is that perhaps a child ought at some stage to have the option of knowing who its genetic parent is (a principle now accepted in the case of adopted children). This may be a persuasive consideration against anonymity, although it may call for reconsideration of the worry about bringing in a third party. Victor finds himself feeling very uneasy with the thought of their child's perhaps later seeking out the identity of the genetic father, though he realizes that adoptive parents also have to face this worry. All things considered, Mary and Victor are content with the current arrangement whereby there is donor anonymity. The issue concerning information about donors is one we return to below.

9.3 *IN VITRO* FERTILIZATION

While artificial insemination is not particularly novel or modern, although techniques are constantly being refined, *in vitro* fertilization (IVF) certainly is. Put very simply, *in vitro* fertilization involves removing a ripe egg from a woman and in a glass (*in vitro*) mixing it with some semen so that fertilization takes place. Fertilization takes place *in vitro* as opposed to natural fertilization in the body (*in vivo*). After successful fertilization, the resulting embryo is then transferred to a woman's uterus where it is hoped it will implant and subsequently develop. In practice, given the problems of achieving a successful fertilization and a subsequent successful implantation, more than one egg is fertilized and more than one embryo is transferred to the womb. This does mean a risk of a multiple pregnancy.

In what situations might IVF be used? First of all, if tubal surgery has not corrected a previous difficulty with the fallopian tubes, IVF allows the possibility of overcoming this problem by bypassing the tubes. A child born in such circumstances is, like a child born after AIH, the genetic child of both partners. Second, if a woman cannot produce an egg, an egg or eggs could be donated by a donor, fertilized *in vitro* with her male partner's semen and transferred into her uterus. Egg donation is the female equivalent of semen donation. In this case, any child subsequently born is genetically related only to the male partner. Third, if both partners are infertile, eggs and semen could be donated, fertilized *in vitro*, and the resulting embryo transferred into the female partner's uterus. Embryo donation has been described by Warnock (1984, p. 40) as constituting 'a form of prenatal adoption, with the advantage over normal adoption that the couple share the experience of pregnancy and childbirth'.

In the case of Mary and Victor, we noted some considerations that might be taken to count against AID. The same considerations might also be taken to count against IVF and the egg and embryo donation which it makes possible. These may not in the end be compelling reasons, but a deliberating couple would need to take account of them. However, perhaps there is also a moral objection to the very idea of donating either semen or egg. It might be thought that is wrong because gametes have a special significance as the 'seed of life'. On the other hand, if such gametes are not going to be used by their donors to produce life, perhaps considerations of respect for life favour their getting an opportunity to become a human person. The stark choice here is between no life and one or more extra lives.

It must also be acknowledged that some individuals could not rest content knowing that, possibly, there exists a child genetically related to them with whom no relationship is possible. As we saw (in section 8.12, above), the very thought of that can lead some individuals to demand from abortion the death of the foetus. However it is not obvious that everyone should feel like this. And the continuing existence of donors and of women who are prepared to allow their children to be adopted suggests that not everyone does.

In connection with the anonymity of semen donors, we asked what information should be given to the couple receiving the donation and decided to defer our answer until later. We shall examine this issue now.

The Warnock *Report* (1984, p. 24) recommended that, in keeping with the desire to protect the anonymity of all parties, information given to the couple requiring the donation should be restricted to information about genetic health and ethnic group. Why should the information given be so limited? Warnock (1984, p. 24) was of the opinion that

> as a matter of principle we do not wish to encourage the possibility of prospective parents seeking donors with specific characteristics by the use of whose semen they hope to give birth to a particular type of child. We do not therefore want detailed descriptions of donors to be used as a basis for choice, but we believe that the couple should be given sufficient relevant information for their reassurance.

(The same would hold for egg as for semen donation.)

But why should the information, limited as it is, centre on genetic health and ethnic origin and why should this be thought to reassure? Warnock (1984) appears to be of the opinion that this information will be of some universal import, of much wider relevance than the choices which represent mere desires or wants of individual prospective parents. However, we should note that some parents are quite happy to adopt handicapped babies. Further, assuming that the information about ethnic origin is given to enable parents to choose to have a donor of their own ethnic group, we must also note that many parents who adopt are quite happy to adopt children who belong to a different ethnic group. However, to take just knowledge of the ethnic group, it may be, in the case of AID parents, that this information is crucial for them. It is hard to see how this could be other than racist. If this is the ground for making available information about donors' ethnic groups, it could not be easily defended. However, Warnock (1984, p. 25) provided one possible line of non-racist justification in its discussion of AID parents.

As matters stand at present there is a temptation for the couple to conceal the true situation when a child is conceived as a result of AID in order to hide the fact that the husband is infertile and to avoid unfavourable reaction among relatives and friends.

AID parents may seek to protect their child from being made to feel different from other children. Again, very often infertility is incorrectly taken to signify a lack of sexual potency. For at least those reasons (and there may be others), couples may wish to conceal just how a child has been conceived. Certainly secrecy or confidentiality could be lost if the prospective parents were not given reassurances concerning the donor's ethnic origin. However, many other physical features and mental and intellectual traits also have a basis in heredity. These too could lead to loss of secrecy. So the need to guarantee secrecy would indicate the provision of much more information. This could be done without compromising the anonymity of the donor.

It might, however, be argued that this is unfair as ethnic differences are plainly visible while other character traits and features are not so prominent. Moreover, it is not uncommon for individuals to comment on those traits and features and to remark how unlike some members of a family are, and where the children are genetically both parents' such comments are not taken as threatening. Nevertheless, the very same comments may well be perceived as threatening in the case of AID families. There a greater sensitivity might be experienced, and remarks that a child looks different may cause intense unease and embarrassment. If this is so, and Warnock (1984) has acknowledged the sensitivity, this would reinforce the case for more information being made available.

With regard to both semen and egg donation, Warnock (1984, pp. 25, 37–38) argued that any such donation should be absolute and that, in consequence, all so-called parental rights and duties should be forfeited by the donor. In particular, in the case of egg donation, this would mean that the woman giving birth should be regarded in law as the mother. We shall enquire whether there are circumstances where this might be questioned, such as in the case of surrogacy arrangements.

9.4 SURROGACY

Surrogacy occurs when a woman agrees to carry a foetus to term for a couple, and, when the child is born, to hand it over to them. Surrogacy is not new; instances of surrogacy can be found in the Old Testament. What is new, however, is that with the help of AID or IVF the surrogate mother does not need to have sexual relations with any man. Why should any person seek to secure the services of a surrogate mother?

The reasons could be medical or nonmedical. In the medical case, surrogacy would be of value if a woman had no uterus, or if pregnancy was life-threatening or if she had found it difficult to establish a pregnancy. In all these cases, the woman may, or may not, be able to produce healthy eggs. In the nonmedical case, a woman may simply desire another woman to endure the discomfort, as she sees it, of pregnancy and may, or may not, be willing to have her egg used.

In the more usual medical case, a couple may see surrogacy as the only method available to them to obtain a child which is at the very least the genetic child of the male partner. In such cases, AID is often used to establish the pregnancy, but the surrogate mother supplies the egg and the subsequent child is genetically hers. In other cases, the egg may be supplied to the surrogate mother by the woman requiring help and with the aid of IVF, using the semen of the woman's male partner, the pregnancy will be established. In such a case, a child born is genetically the commissioning couple's; the surrogate mother has merely engaged in 'womb leasing' (Glover *et al.*, 1989, p. 67).

It may be thought that if such individuals desire a child so much, adoption would suffice. First of all, there are not sufficient 'normal' babies to be adopted to satisfy the demand. Second, and probably more important, what such couples desire, and surrogacy would give them, is to have a child genetically related to at least one of them. Being a 'natural' father or mother seems to be important.

And yet what does it mean to say that an individual is a genetic or natural father or mother? It means that someone else carries genetic material from that individual. It means nothing more than this. The fact of genetic parenthood is a very brute fact. In as much as it is merely genetic, the relationship of a human child to its genetic parents is exactly the same as the relationship of, say, a cuckoo chick to its genetic parents. All we think of as warm and tender and caring, etc., in parent–child relationships attaches to social and not to genetic parenthood. Of course, normally, genetic and social links are present, and fathers and mothers share both. But with adoption, and now with the development of AID, IVF, egg and embryo donation, we are being forced to recognize that genetic and social links need not be intermingled within one concept of parenthood. Is an individual less of a parent if there is no genetic link to the child?

These are undoubtedly difficult questions. But there is a case for thinking that the concepts of parenthood, father and mother are best analysed in terms of social roles which the individuals concerned play. Genetic links on their own make an individual neither a better nor a worse father or mother. Still, we must recognize that for many individuals it is important to be a parent to children which are genetically their own. For many, semen or egg donation would always be ruled out because they could not countenance 'their' children existing in the world but not parented by them (cf. sections 8.12 and 9.3, above). But, while we recognize this fact, if what we ultimately value is individuals being good parents, good fathers and mothers, we can agree that such individuals can exist even when the genetic link to their children is absent. Thus, if a surrogacy arrangement is sought solely to allow the possibility of genetic parenthood, it is not at all clear that this is an end worth striving for.

Would such a conclusion also count against support being given to some of the other techniques for alleviating infertility? It might, but it depends on whether the end to be achieved is disproportionate with the means used. In the case of surrogacy, one reason for not permitting it as an option is the possibility of the exploitation of the surrogate mother. Another reason is the existence of 'contracts' which come uncomfortably close to treating babies as merchandise. Depending on how weighty these considerations are, they may tip the balance to such an extent that the end to be achieved does not merit the means used.

This may be seen, if we examine a Warnock (1984) recommendation, referred to previously (section 9.3), that all donation of semen and eggs should be absolute and, in particular, that a woman having received a donated egg and given birth should be regarded as the mother of the child. Could such a proposal hold in the case of surrogacy?

In such a case, if an egg were donated, it would not be a gift or an absolute donation, but rather donated with the idea in mind that any subsequent child would be handed over to the commissioning couple. In such a case, the woman giving birth (the surrogate) would not be regarded as the mother of the child. This seems fair (much more so than if the surrogate mother were the genetic mother because then no donation would have been made) and contracts might exist to reinforce the claim. But what if the surrogate mother refuses to hand over the child? Would the nature of the donation and the existence of contracts be decisive here in forcing a response? What if the woman who donated the egg claimed that her baby was being stolen? Would this be a decisive consideration? On the one hand, the commissioning mother does seem to have a legitimate claim, yet on the other hand, perhaps a baby ought not to be removed from the woman who has carried it to term and given birth even though the egg it developed from is not her own. We feel forced to ask, 'What is the point of this arrangement?'

If the point is merely to allow individuals to acquire children to whom they are genetically related, our earlier discussion prompts the question whether the end warrants the difficulties and problems involved in the means. Of course not all surrogacy agreements need end in tears; however, a significant number have and, in the light of this, a solution is perhaps to be sought not in the introduction of legally binding contracts, which may in practice be unenforceable, but rather in a closer look at what partners to surrogacy agreements are hoping to achieve. Genetic or partial genetic parenthood may not seem worth using another individual for (and it is not merely the use of a womb), with all the emotional trauma involved, for a substantial period of time.

9.5 EMBRYO EXPERIMENTATION

IVF was developed through embryo experimentation. The discussion which often takes place as to its moral acceptability often ignores this fact and assumes that we are being asked whether it would be a good thing to allow such experimentation or research in the near future. What in fact we are being asked is whether there are good moral reasons to allow it to continue.

What has been and what could be achieved by researching on embryos? First of all, as already stated, embryo research has allowed the development of IVF because it was only through experimentation on the very early embryo that such a technique to alleviate certain cases of infertility came to be possible. However, IVF is not at present particularly successful; it does not guarantee a baby at the end of the procedure, and researchers are convinced that it is only by allowing further and continuing research that the success rate can be improved. Second, it is believed that such research will enable advances to be made in discovering the causes of infertility in general, miscarriages and, most importantly, genetic disorders. Much is made of the last claim because it is widely believed that the elimination of genetic disorders will be universally welcomed. What is promised here is threefold: at the very least, and initially, the possibility of screening 'at risk' embryos – leading to abortion if they are affected; using IVF, putting back into the woman only embryos which are free of the disorder; and, as research develops, the possibility of the replacement of defective genes in the affected embryo itself, which would remove the need either to abort or to discard affected embryos.

Such ends may seem laudable, so why is there extensive public disquiet? In the case of research conducted on adult humans, it is necessary to obtain the consent of research subjects before research can commence and, while it cannot be guaranteed, there is often the possibility that the research will be of some direct benefit to them. In the case of embryos, such conditions cannot be satisfied. Consent obviously cannot be sought, and embryos researched on are discarded subsequently. As opponents of such research might put it, they are not given the chance to realize their potential.

This concern for the well-being of embryos may seem out of place in societies which condone abortion, legislate for it, and, in the case of Great Britain, permit it up to 24 weeks after conception. After all, the research which is proposed would take place on the very early embryo. If indeed the death of foetuses is acceptable, why should research on and the subsequent death of very early embryos pose an acute ethical dilemma?

Consider the following argument:

Death is the greatest evil that can happen to an individual.
Research, while it may be wrong, cannot be as great an evil as death.
So, if it is morally permissible to kill foetuses up to 24 weeks after conception, it must also be morally permissible to conduct research on early embryos.

Three responses can be made to this line of thought. First, it is commonly thought that death is in many cases a merciful release from states that are worse than death. So the first premiss is false. Second, it is the case that abortion is not universally approved of and those who oppose it would be of the opinion that to conduct research on embryos further devalues their status and enhances societal approval of abortion. Research would not be conducted on young children or adults without consent no matter how great the benefit. So if it is permitted on embryos it reinforces their inferior position. Third, even those who morally approve of abortion might feel that additional considerations apply when considering the moral permissibility of research. Research, for example, might cause the embryo to experience pain and could be supported morally only if the embryo has not developed sufficiently to experience pain or is adequately anaesthetized.

Two possible reasons for opposing embryo experimentation are that the embryo has moral standing and that it can experience pain. If these reasons cannot be ultimately sustained then, in view of the suggested benefits, there would appear to be a persuasive case in favour of embryo experimentation.

The Warnock *Report* (1984) considered this topic and among the members there was majority support in favour of such research. Warnock (1984, pp. 63–64) believed that while the embryo should be offered some legal protection, this must not be thought of as absolute protection.

That protection should exist does not entail that this protection may not be waived in certain specific circumstances. Having examined the evidence presented to us about the types of research which might be carried out on human embryos produced in vitro, the majority of us hold that such research should not be totally prohibited. . . . Nevertheless, . . . such research must be subject to stringent controls and monitoring.

The proposal produced was that research could be conducted on embryos only up to fourteen days after conception. This proposal that fourteen days is acceptable seems to have won near-universal approval from all those who approve of and are engaged in such research. In truth, nothing of any great significance occurs at fourteen days in the life of the embryo, except that prior to this time it is not possible to know how many embryos are in fact present or to differentiate the developing embryo or embryos from the placenta and the other life-support systems, all of which are part of the greater cell mass.

Some writers refer to the pre-fourteen day embryo as a pre-embryo. This, we think, is confusing and reflects an attempt to make embryo research appear more acceptable by suggesting that real embryos are not actually involved. Embryos, however, do not suddenly come into existence at this time. (For discussion see Holland, 1990.) Certainly, at fourteen days there is no possibility of pain or distress being experienced by the embryo; but it must be stressed that fourteen days was not chosen for this specific reason. Avoidance of pain would have permitted a much later date.

One other issue considered by Warnock (1984) concerned how embryos were acquired for research purposes. As we have seen in our discussion of IVF, given the difficulties involved more than one egg is normally fertilized and more than one embryo subsequently transferred into the woman. However, more embryos may be produced than are required for one particular treatment. Such embryos are known as spare embryos and a problem can arise as to what you do with them.

Some members of the Warnock (1984) committee felt that it would be appropriate to use such spare embryos and not any other embryos for research purposes. Embryos specifically created for research or obtained by other means were not acceptable research subjects.

> These members argue that it cannot be consonant with the special status that the Inquiry as a whole has agreed should be afforded to the human embryo, to cause it to exist, yet to allow it no possibility of implantation. Similarly others argue that it is fertilization itself that is unique and it ought not to be undertaken when there is no chance whatever that the potential for human development will be fulfilled.
>
> (Warnock, 1984, p. 67)

Is there a morally justifiable distinction here? Are spare embryos the only appropriate research subjects? First of all, these same members of the committee did feel able to accept IVF, from a moral perspective, as an acceptable means of treating infertility and it is because of how the treatments are carried out that spare embryos exist. To condone IVF is to accept the fertilization of eggs where from a statistical point of view it is known that a certain number of embryos will be given no possibility of implantation. Of course when eggs are fertilized for IVF treatment, it is not known at the moment of fertilization which or how many subsequent embryos will be implanted. It may certainly be the intention, if necessary, to implant all. But it must also be known that the statistical probability is that only a few will be implanted and for the rest 'there is no chance whatever that the potential for human development will be fulfilled.' Thus these same members of the committee to be consistent must also reject IVF treatment as well, or, if they do not, find a new basis for their argument that a clear moral distinction exists between the use of these differently generated embryos in research.

Recently, with improved techniques of freezing, the problem of what to do with spare embryos is not as pressing as it once was. They can be stored to be used again at a subsequent treatment, if that is necessary. Thus an argument to the effect that only spare embryos are suitable research subjects would severely curtail further research work, and would be effectively an argument against research as such.

Moreover, if it is morally permissible to conduct research on some embryos, it must be morally permissible to conduct it on other embryos unless there are good and convincing reasons why not. Embryos do not have to be researched on. If being researched on is appropriate it must be because of the value accorded to such research. The majority view of the Warnock committee (1984, p. 69) was to endorse research 'on any embryo resulting from in vitro fertilization, whatever its provenance.'

9.6 GENETIC ENGINEERING

This is a very large topic demanding extensive treatment. Here we shall briefly discuss one or two issues.

Embryo research opens up the possibility that certain genetic disorders could eventually be eliminated from our species. When one reflects on the nature of some of these disorders and their devastating effect on the sufferers and their families, this can only be approved of. Such 'negative' genetic engineering, as it is commonly called, seems most welcome, indeed as welcome as the elimination of cancer would be. Genetic manipulation to eliminate disorders is viewed as a good thing.

However, the manipulation of genes could be deployed to improve the human gene pool. Such 'positive' genetic manipulation to improve, for example, intelligence, artistic ability and athletic prowess is not generally viewed as a good thing. Indeed it is viewed by many people with horror, conjuring up images of mad scientists creating monsters or malign politicians indulging in eugenics or designing people who can be easily manipulated for the politician's own ends.

But would it necessarily be a bad thing if we were all more intelligent, more musical, etc.? One general response is that this would not be unwelcome but the fear of the unknown price to pay is what deters many individuals. For genes may be changed to improve intelligence, but there may be a consequent increase in other character traits which would not be so welcome. Fear of the unknown is what deters here. But if fear of unknown effects is a reason for opposition to 'positive' genetic engineering then it is also a reason for opposing 'negative' genetic engineering.

Furthermore, is there a sharp distinction between 'positive' and 'negative' genetic engineering? Both are concerned with changing people. The reasons are perhaps different. But what both seek is improvement: improvement with the disappearance of genetic disorders and improvement with the enhancement of certain normally admired characteristics. A world in which genetic disorders did not exist and in which there existed people who were more intelligent, athletic, musical, etc. would seem to be a better world than one in which genetic disorders only had been eliminated with no further improvement in the positive characteristics of the population. Some reason needs to be given for the different societal responses to the two allegedly distinct forms of genetic engineering (for a comprehensive discussion of the issues, see Glover, 1984).

TEN

Death, dying and easing death

My personal interest is history, especially the history of the Second War, and of how it is possible the way dictatorships get the people behind them. Dictatorship has not gone away, it is still with us in the world, and it comes when people force their ideas onto other people. Once it was the Catholic Church persecuting those who did not think like them; and the Nazis the same, then South Africa, or Pinochet. We are talking about the rights of the patient, and the deep right of choosing the moment when you want to die, and doing this in a private relation with your doctor. I think many of our critics are projecting their own death-problems onto the patient. When you force your ethical ideas or your view of what is pathological onto other people, against their will – then that is opening the door to Auschwitz.
(Dr Theo van Berkestijn, a Dutch doctor and supporter of Voluntary Euthanasia)

The duty of medicine is to protect the patient against the egoism of the healthy. I use the example of the Nazi programme because it is the only clear one available. And I say that the euthanasia now practised in Holland is opening the door to the same mentality, opening the door to Auschwitz.
(Dr Andre Wynen, a survivor of a German concentration camp and Secretary General of the World Medical Association)

As can be observed from the above quotations (from an article entitled 'Life or Death?' in the *Guardian* newspaper, 17 February 1988), a discussion of hastening or delaying death can connect with powerful and deeply felt convictions. A person may see denying the right of a patient to choose an early death as constraining human choice in the way charac-

teristic of authoritarian societies. On the other hand one may also fear
that a society which condones euthanasia will so weaken respect for human
life that mass killings for a variety of reasons will become a real possibility.
Holland is such a society; there physicians can avoid legal prosecution for
voluntary euthanasia provided it is carried out in accordance with established guidelines. Meanwhile nurses resuscitating a patient often find themselves wondering 'Why are we doing this? Whose benefit is it for? Is this
the kind of care we should be giving?'

10.1 DEATH AND DYING

There are few certainties in life, but one which we all, to varying degrees,
try to come to terms with is our own death. For some, death is not a
problem, the subject of an existential concern, rather it is the process of
dying and in particular whether that process is free from pain and trauma
('Death is not an event in life: we do not live to experience death. . . .',
Wittgenstein, 1961, 6.4311). For others, death and with it the possible
end of all conscious experiences is the major concern, and solace may be
sought and found in the claims of certain religions that death is not the
terminus of life but merely the vehicle which facilitates new and qualitatively different experiences all of which are attributable to a continuing
subject of experience.

Be that as it may, we all would like to die well. However, different
people make contrasting judgements of personal value about death. For
some, dying well is dying a quick, unexpected death. For others, it might
be dying in such a way that one can appropriately arrange one's affairs
and take one's leave of family and friends and accept death with a certain
equanimity. What will be commonly accepted is the desirability of avoiding
a process of dying which is extended, painful and traumatic, and where
one may feel that one is a burden to loved ones and where the nature of
the dying is such that it poses a threat to fundamental human dignity.
Many of us could tell a story of horror which may, for example, be derived
from witnessing the unpleasant death of a loved one or observing the slow
fade into oblivion of friends with senile dementia.

The question is, how does one achieve a 'good' death given the level
of suffering that is present in the world? One response to this is to seek
to make the process of dying a better one. This response is the basic motive
of the hospice movement. We return to this below. Another response is
to argue that human persons must be permitted to take their own life or
have their life terminated by others if it is perceived to be in their own
interests. In other words, they should have the options of committing
suicide or receiving euthanasia. We shall proceed to discuss these topics
after briefly reviewing the relations between law, morality and euthanasia.

10.2 MORALITY AND LAW

Euthanasic killing is illegal. Up until 1961, it was illegal to attempt suicide, and assisting a suicide is still illegal. The fact that something is legal does not make it morally right. It might be legal simply because a law making it illegal would be unenforceable or would result in matters being even worse. (Thus an argument for abortion's being legal in the past has been that legalizing it reduces the number of back street abortions; and an argument for prostitution's being legal has been that legalizing it makes easier the control of sexually transmitted diseases.) And the fact that something is illegal does not mean that it is morally wrong. Harbouring Jews in the later years of the Third Reich was illegal yet not immoral. Certain kinds of interracial marriage were for many years illegal in South Africa, yet they were surely not immoral. Thus something's being legal does not make it morally right and something's being illegal does not make it morally wrong.

Nevertheless, it is reasonable to hope that a system of laws will coincide with morality to a great extent, so that to a great extent things which are legal are also morally right and things which are illegal are also morally wrong. And, when there is scope for improvement in the match between morality and legality, reasonable people often seek to get laws changed in order to improve the match. Thus people have campaigned on moral grounds to get slavery made illegal, to have capital punishment abolished, to suppress pornography, to legalize suicide, to have abortion made illegal, to have abortion legalized, to have euthanasia legalized, and so on. This is not to say that those who would reform the law on moral grounds are always guaranteed to have the best moral arguments. However, the fact that what they are about can be understood and that laws can be criticized from a moral point of view shows that thinking that something is illegal is not the same as thinking that that thing is morally wrong.

For present purposes, the upshot of this is that the present illegality of euthanasia does not mean that there is no scope for discussing the morality of it. Further, that something is morally right is not always sufficient ground for its being made legal. We shall discuss the morality of suicide and euthanasia in the rest of this chapter, but we shall not address the question of what laws there ought to be.

10.3 SUICIDE

What is suicide? Suicide occurs when an individual determines to kill himself or herself and succeeds in doing so. Suicide is one kind of self-killing; an individual wants or intends to die and brings about the desired death.

From a moral perspective, it might be argued, suicide is wrong because it involves killing, taking or ending a human life, and there is decisive moral reason against all such killing. Many of us would be unable, however, to maintain an absolute no-killing principle, because of a belief that killing can be permissible in such cases as, for example, self-defence, war, just rebellion, and capital punishment. Nevertheless, one influential argument in moral discussions of suicide centres on the significance of the principle of the sanctity of life. Support for such a principle, it is thought, would prevent any qualitative consideration, such as the state of an individual's health, being decisive in determining whether an individual ought to be permitted to end his or her own life. The sanctity of life principle has been argued for from within both religious and secular frameworks, so we shall turn now to examine each in turn.

10.4 A RELIGIOUS PRINCIPLE

It might seem strange that within the Judaeo-Christian tradition the principle of the sanctity of life should be thought important. Within that tradition, what is revered is not life *per se*, but rather *human* life. The tradition teaches that humankind was given 'dominion over the animals'; and, although animals were to be respected as God's creatures, their role was to serve the needs of humankind. This position was reinforced by the ontological claim that humans, and only humans, had immortal souls and were created in the image of their divine maker. So within that religious tradition, the principle of the sanctity of life is really a principle of the sanctity of *human* life.

However, adherence to the principle, so interpreted, does not mean that in general religious believers accept that it is always wrong to take human life. Just war theory and acceptable conditions for a morally correct rebellion had theologians amongst their earliest exponents. Support for capital punishment is not limited to secular moralists. Justifiable killing is certainly accepted. The murder of fellow human beings is disapproved of; this is taken to be an instance of unjustifiable killing. But if this is the case, the principle of the sanctity of human life only extends to include unjustifiable killing and not all killing. Could suicide, as a self-inflicted killing, be acceptable?

In contemplating suicide, an individual may believe that, given the quality of his or her known future existence, death is preferable to continuing to live. Here quality considerations are counted as reasons for killing just as it may be argued that they may be taken as reasons for killing in the context of a just war or a just rebellion. In both cases the projected quality of life – in the one case the life of an individual and in the other the life of a society – may be decisive in determining future action. There seems to be no good reason why considerations of quality should count in one case and not in the other. Thus if killing may be permissible in a just war or rebellion on this basis, there is no reason why suicide should not also be permissible.

Perhaps it is an awareness of this that has led certain religious thinkers to deny that some self-killings, which may be thought of as suicides, are in fact suicides. Self-killings which occur because of qualitative considerations are not suicides because true suicide occurs only when an individual takes her life not because of how things are – how the world or life is treating her – but because she is rejecting the gift of life itself and, of course, God. Some self-killings which are not suicides are performed for the ends to be achieved and are not always wrong; whether they are wrong depends on whether the end to be achieved justifies the means taken. However, where life itself and God are simply rejected, there is no purpose or end to be achieved other than ending one's life. Nevertheless, given the importance of the concept of life as a gift (life being perceived as a gift from God and the recipient of the gift its steward who cannot simply hand it back), it is questionable whether self-killings which are not suicides, or any other kinds of killing, are morally easier to justify than suicide proper. It should be noted that the gift metaphor can also be interpreted in a quite different way, as we often think of a gift as an absolute donation which the receiver is entitled to use in whatever way he or she thinks fit.

This is one central religious position on suicide. Suicide is fundamentally impermissible not merely because it infringes the principle of the sanctity of human life but because it is a rejection of God's gift of life. Indeed whatever strength as a principle the principle of the sanctity of human life has for religious believers derives from the notion that life is a gift from God. As St Thomas Aquinas (1265–1273, Pt. II–II, Q.64, Act. 5, p. 103) said, '..because life is God's gift to man, and is subject to His power . . . it belongs to God alone to pronounce sentence of death and life'. Only God can decide when an individual should die; it is a fundamental sin for an individual to believe that he or she can decide the appropriate moment. The philosopher David Hume (1777, p. 107) showed the untenability of this by pointing out its unacceptable implications:

Were the disposal of human life so much reserved as the peculiar province of the Almighty that it were an encroachment on his right, for men to dispose of their own lives; it would be equally criminal to act for the preservation of life as for its destruction. If I turn aside a stone which is falling upon my head, I disturb the course of nature, and I invade the peculiar province of the Almighty by lengthening out my life beyond the period which by the general laws of matter and motion he had assigned it.

If killing oneself is wrong for the reason given, then preserving life when in danger must also be wrong because the danger faced may be God's way of terminating an existence; God may have decided the individual should die. If suicide is wrong for this reason, then saving or prolonging life can also be wrong for the very same reason.

10.5 SANCTITY OF LIFE: A SECULAR FRAMEWORK

A secular principle of the sanctity of life like a religious one turns out to embody a particular concern for human life and not life *per se*. Even if secular thinkers resist this way of expressing the point, arguing that they do not wish to make a sharp division between humankind and the other animals (and unlike the religious believer they have no ontological basis for doing so), it is quite clear that for them the life of certain animals counts for more, or is of greater value, than the life of other animals. Proponents of a secular sanctity of life principle would agree that, to borrow an old example, if faced with the choice of either saving a cow stranded on a rock by an incoming tide or a human person in a similar predicament, the most rational and morally correct course of action would be to save the human person. And indeed if the choice were between saving a rat and saving a chimpanzee, the chimpanzee would be saved. On what basis can such judgements be justified?

A possible basis for such judgements would be one which referred to the respective qualities of life open to each of the animals in question. It is because the life enjoyed by a human person is thought to be qualitatively superior to the life enjoyed by a cow that the saving of the human person is believed to be required and, for similar considerations, the life of the chimpanzee is preferred to that of the rat. Reference is made to the quality of life enjoyed by each of the species in question.

In making such judgements supporters of a secular sanctity of life principle do not object to the drawing of qualitative distinctions across the divisions between the species. However, while quite willing to draw such qualitative distinctions between the species, they are not prepared to draw such distinctions within the species *Homo sapiens*. Thus, while human persons are qualitatively superior in terms of the quality of the existence or life they enjoy to the level of existence or life enjoyed by a cow, this does not mean that such distinctions count when comparisons are made between the lives of individual members of the species *Homo sapiens*. At that level, qualitative distinctions must be eschewed, and all individuals must be considered simply as individuals whose lives must be protected even from themselves no matter what level of pain or anguish they are suffering. This is what a secular principle of the sanctity of human life demands (and it is a principle of the sanctity of *human* life).

Can such a principle be defended? First of all, why should human life be treated in this special fashion? How can drawing this cordon around human life be justified in a secular way? It will be recalled that, for the religious believer, there is a real ontological difference between human-kind and the animals; for the secular moralist no such difference exists. All that does exist in nature are different species with differing capacities. If life is to be respected, why must it only be human life which is accorded this absolute respect? If it is the quality of life which humans can achieve which is decisive in according them absolute protection, why must humans who do not have the potential to achieve that quality of life – or who are in the process of either losing it or have already lost it – also receive absolute protection? It would seem that it is only by tacitly relying on a religious frame of reference that such reasoning could make any sense. Second, once this is recognized, qualitative considerations will be seen to be relevant not only to distinctions drawn between species but also to legitimate concerns about the level of existence endured by certain human beings. Then, in the absence of good reason for embracing a sanctity of life principle, it seems wiser not to accept it as offering a clear guide to informed thought on these questions.

10.6 SUICIDE: A RIGHT TO DIE?

We entered into our discussion of the sanctity of life principle, in both its religious and secular forms, because it is sometimes thought that such a principle decisively rules suicide out and removes the need for further enquiry. As we have now seen, it cannot be assumed that further enquiry is superfluous. It will, we hope, become clearer that quality of life considerations are centrally relevant to the morality of suicide. It is sometimes said that everyone has a right to die. Often what is meant is a right to die at a time of one's own choice. The principle of autonomy seems to support such a right.

But perhaps this does not settle the matter. Perhaps suicide attempts indicate not a wish to die but a level of mental instability which would call into question the rationality of the person's judgements. Is a person who attempts suicide, to speak colloquially, really sane? Now it is certainly true that many individuals who attempt suicide may do so for a variety of reasons: it may simply be a cry for help; it may be a ridiculous response to a very trivial problem; it may be an ill thought-out response to a very serious problem or it may be a considered response to a situation which seems to demand this solution. What is important is to avoid the temptation to generalize. Some individual suicides may be mentally ill, others may be confused and frightened, still others will be extremely rational and know exactly what they hope to achieve. The desire to die is not always expressive of some deep, pathological irrationality.

Given the respect we must hold for human autonomy, this means that, just as there are occasions when we shall fight to retain a human life because that is what the individual wants, so there will also have to be occasions when out of respect for what the individual wants we shall have to stand by and observe a life being extinguished. The Catholic Linacre report (1982, p. 45) notes in a section entitled 'The legal right to refuse treatment':

> It is clear that the doctor must respect the mature and sufficiently lucid patient's refusal of treatment even if he disapproves of that refusal, believing, in a life-threatening situation, that it is tantamount to suicide. In respecting that refusal the doctor is respecting the patient's autonomy.

Linacre, however, while recognizing the patient's autonomy in such a situation, denies that a suicidal intention is in any circumstances morally acceptable; and the Suicide Act of 1961 prevents a doctor in any circumstances facilitating a suicide. However, an Institute of Medical Ethics Working Party report (1990, p. 613.) came to the conclusion that

> to prolong life which a person, being of sound mind, does not wish to have prolonged, contradicts the fundamental moral principle of respect for autonomy and, in some cases, the doctor's duty to relieve suffering. A patient's sustained wish to die is a sufficient reason for a doctor to allow him to do so.

Human autonomy must be the bedrock on which the right to commit suicide rests, and the rationality of the judgement made by any individual committing suicide will depend on the reasons that individual has for acting in that fashion. The moral status of the action will likewise depend on those reasons. In certain cases, the 'reasons' will be such as to manifest a serious mental instability which rules out moral appraisal of the action. In other cases, the reasons may be such as to amount to the individual's simply 'running away' from serious problems and rejecting suicide would have been the more morally courageous course. In yet other cases, the reasons may include the individual's projected quality of life being such that one can only sympathize with the suicide. There is no definitive moral judgement covering all cases. An important issue remains the projected quality of life for that individual and the individual assessment of that quality.

10.7 EUTHANASIA: DEFINITION AND VARIANTS

Suicide involves an individual taking his or her own life; in the case of euthanasia another individual does the killing. This fact, coupled with the 'bad press' euthanasia has received by being associated with the Nazis (as exemplified in one of our opening quotations), has led many people to be very wary of the concept. It is one thing to accept suicide on the grounds of respect for human autonomy, but euthanasia raises difficult and complex issues. Perhaps the best way to begin our discussion is to formulate a definition of euthanasia and distinguish between different cases.

Euthanasia is sometimes simply referred to as mercy killing. While there is often virtue in simplicity, in this case a more detailed and explanatory definition is required. In employing the term 'euthanasia', we are referring to the intentional killing of individuals whose mental or physical state or both is such that it is believed that it would be in their best interests to die. Note that these individuals are killed because it is believed that it would be in their best interests to die; the interests of the person doing the killing are not the dominant feature of the situation as would be the case when an individual is simply murdered because it is in the best interests of the murderer that he or she die. This is what is distinctive about euthanasia and explains why such killings are often qualified as mercy killings.

10.8 VOLUNTARY EUTHANASIA

Voluntary euthanasia occurs when an individual is killed at his or her own request. An individual, because of a distressing state, desires an end to his or her life and, being of sound mind, requests another individual, normally a doctor, to terminate his or her existence. The individual concerned may not be able to commit suicide nor indeed have the expertise to do so, but it is assumed that if that ability and expertise were present then the individual would commit suicide. Unless that assumption is present, doubt will be cast on the voluntary nature of the euthanasia.

As such, voluntary euthanasia differs from *assisted suicide* where another individual provides the means by which the individual committing suicide dies but does not perform the actual killing.

Respect for individual autonomy and the right of an individual to choose in distressing circumstances the time of death provide *prima facie* grounds in support of voluntary euthanasia.

10.9 NONVOLUNTARY EUTHANASIA

Nonvoluntary euthanasia occurs when an individual is killed even though it is not possible to ascertain his or her view on the death. A doctor, in consultation with an immediate family and the health care team, may judge that it would be in the best interests of the individual to die. Such instances of euthanasia could include, *inter alia*, the infanticide of handicapped infants such as, for example, spina bifida or Down's syndrome babies, and the withdrawal of life-support facilities or other treatment from individuals who are utterly dependent on them and who have been severely brain damaged. In cases of the latter kind we may have some idea of the individuals' previously expressed views on euthanasia, and on what treatment or nontreatment they might think appropriate for them in the kind of situation they are now in.

Nonvoluntary euthanasia raises in an acute form the question of the legitimacy of making quality of life judgements about the life of another individual and on that basis deciding to terminate a life.

10.10 INVOLUNTARY EUTHANASIA

Involuntary euthanasia would occur if an individual were to be killed, even though he has not been consulted or is known not to want to die. The following would be such a case: a doctor decides that because of an individual's condition death is in his or her best interests; but the doctor does not consider it appropriate to consult the individual about this decision, or does consult the individual and encounters a negative reaction but still decides to kill the individual. Insofar as euthanasia is supposed to be concerned with the interests of the individual to be killed, what better spokesperson of that interest could there be than the individual who is the subject of the judgement? In such a serious matter, paternalism cannot be allowed to undermine autonomy. Indeed there can be no serious moral debate concerning the moral legitimacy of involuntary euthanasia in health care.

The *prima facie* grounds we identified for supporting voluntary euthanasia would definitively count against any measure of support for involuntary euthanasia.

10.11 ACTIVE AND PASSIVE EUTHANASIA

All the kinds of euthanasia we have described could be brought about in one of two ways: either active means could be taken to end a life, for example, by the administering of a lethal injection, or passive means could be used to end a life by withholding readily available treatment such as drugs or life-support equipment. In the first case, a person is killed; in the second case, a person is allowed to die. Many of those who endorse euthanasia favour active means for moral reasons; others see a moral equivalence between active and passive means, while still others morally favour passive means. Other people who oppose euthanasia can however see some merit in not inflicting aggressive treatment on certain patients or in withholding treatment even though as a result death may be hastened. They would stress that their acquiescence in the resulting death is not participation in a euthanasic act.

10.12 THE MORALITY OF VOLUNTARY EUTHANASIA

Mary is a 78-year-old widow whose family have not merely left home but lost contact altogether with their mother. Last year Mary was diagnosed as suffering from bone cancer, and despite all the best efforts of the health care team it has proved very difficult to control her pain. She is now feeling very distressed and, being constantly in pain, can see little point to her life. Joan, the nurse who has been in most contact with her, believing that Mary lacks companionship and feels that no one cares, has tried unsuccessfully to develop a meaningful relationship with her. Mary's condition is continuing to deteriorate and no analgesia is adequate. A few days ago when Joan approached her, Mary, who has always known about her condition and prognosis, asked tentatively whether the doctors could 'end it all'. Joan took this as a sign that she must make even greater efforts to cultivate the relationship, but to no avail. In fact, Mary's requests simply became more frequent and more demanding. . . .

As we have seen, voluntary euthanasia occurs when someone is killed at their own request because of their present or projected physical or mental condition. A person is killed because it is believed to be in her or his best interests to die.

The voluntary nature of the killing conceptually positions this form of euthanasia close to suicide. In both cases, a person chooses to die; however, in euthanasia, someone else has to do the killing. If respect for autonomy may lead one to countenance suicide, does this mean that an equal respect for autonomy might lead one to countenance voluntary euthanasia?

Here there is a factor akin to autonomy but pulling in the opposite direction. An autonomous person takes her own decisions. In virtue of this kindred factor, she will also tend to implement them herself unless there is good reason to leave implementation to others. Now, on the one hand, one might feel that if the individual is so desirous of death because of the situation she finds herself in, then it is best if she personally brings about her own death and commits suicide. Why involve a third party in an action which has such serious consequences if the same end can be achieved without that involvement? Respect for autonomy does not point more to euthanasia than to suicide. On the other hand, most people in such horrific situations lack the technical knowledge and drugs required to terminate quickly and painlessly their lives; others may be so totally paralysed that even if they had the knowledge and drugs it would be physically impossible for them to commit suicide. For those lacking knowledge and/or drugs, respect for autonomy would, other things being equal, suggest that a suitably qualified person, provided that he/she accepts the rationality of the judgement, may provide either or both and thus assist in the suicide which the individual wants. For the quadriplegic, respect for autonomy would, other things being equal, suggest that euthanasia should be provided where the quadriplegic believes it is in his best interests. (Whether this places an obligation on a particular group is another question.)

This is what a respect for autonomy would license. As Theo van Berkestijn claimed in the quotation with which we began this chapter, 'We are talking about the rights of the patient, and the deep right of choosing the moment when you want to die, and doing this in a private relation with your doctor'. However, unlike van Berkestijn, we believe that respect for this 'deep right' would in most cases not sanction voluntary euthanasia but merely lead to an acquiescence in an individual's suicide or the provision of the means by which an individual commits suicide, in other words sanction assisted suicide. Voluntary euthanasia would be sanctioned in certain cases, like the one already mentioned, but it would be a relatively rare occurrence.

We adopt this view because we cherish human life. It is precisely because each human life is normally so precious, so worth sustaining, that if a decision is taken to end it the action to do so ought to be performed normally by the individual who has taken that decision. It is hard to see why it should be ended by someone else. What possible purpose could this serve other than to leave the individual who has killed someone else in such circumstances with the lingering doubt as to whether the person killed really wanted to die if he could not bring himself to end his own life? He would constantly be questioning the voluntary nature of this voluntary euthanasia.

However it is hard to deny that there are circumstances, like the instance indicated, where voluntary euthanasia may be permissible from a moral point of view. Such cases are best thought of as proxy suicides, simply because the individual who wants to die would kill himself if he were physically able to do so. The reasons one would have to countenance a suicide or assist a suicide would have to suffice here to commit an act of voluntary euthanasia. Not to do so would abandon such an individual to the imprisonment of his own physical immobility. (For a more detailed treatment, see Glover, 1977, pp. 182–189.)

For some, what respect for autonomy indicates may appear too radical; it may appear to run counter to a health care ethos which is committed to preserving lives at all costs even if individual patients do not want their lives preserved. But surely, in the circumstances envisaged, such an ethos would run the risk of undermining one very good reason there is for respecting human life, namely that human persons are reflective autonomous agents. If there is deliberate neglect or overriding of the wishes of these autonomous agents – which in this case are for their lives not to be preserved – then the respect one has for human life cannot be based on any respect for human autonomy. Respect for human life, in that case, and the desire to preserve it at all costs, cannot be embedded in an ethics to which human personhood and autonomy are central. However, as noted in section 10.2, it is one thing to make a moral case and quite another to make a legal case.

For others, the alteration to the nature of health care provision would be so radical as to count against what has been said. However, true caring may require not merely preserving life at all costs but helping patients in frightfully difficult situations to actualize what for them is the best choice. There may be another possible approach to this problem, and this we shall now discuss.

10.13 GOOD DYING AND THE HOSPICE MOVEMENT

'I'm sorry. There is nothing more we can do.'

Although good doctors avoid writing a patient off in this way, medicine often features in the popular imagination as being concerned above all with curing people. And, to the extent that health care is dominated by medicine, there is a tendency to suppose that the real work of health care is finished when a cure is ruled out. The hospice movement has sought to give the lie to all this and to make noncurative care the main focus of its work.

For many, the thoughts developed in section 10.12 are too defeatist. Dr Cicely Saunders has argued:

> All those who work with dying people are anxious that what is known already should be developed and extended and that terminal care everywhere should become so good that no one need ever ask for voluntary euthanasia.

> (Quoted in Glover, 1977, p. 182.)

Dr Saunders has been associated with the development of the hospice movement which aims to care adequately for terminally ill patients in hospices (see Saunders *et al.*, 1981; and Saunders and Baines, 1989). It is the view of those who are engaged in this work that for far too long a period terminally ill patients in ordinary hospitals did not have their needs catered for, in particular the need for proper control of the pain which they were experiencing. As a consequence, many of these patients sought euthanasia.

Hospice supporters believe that in their special units which cater for all the needs of the dying, including the proper control of pain, requests for euthanasia are no longer common; indeed, if such a request is made, it is perceived as a defeat of their method. To permit euthanasia, it is thought, is to accept a second-best solution to the problem. Moreover, by removing the problem it would also remove the pressure for the development of better and more adequate care of the dying.

This is a difficult problem. On the one hand, it is plausible to suppose that prohibiting voluntary euthanasia will keep up the pressure for adequate care of the dying much as prohibiting private health care and private schools would create pressure for high standards in the national health service and in the state education system. On the other hand, the benign effects of such pressure always take time to come about; and, in the meantime, not only is individual choice curtailed but also the individuals whose plight is the source of pressure suffer disadvantage.

The achievements of the hospice movement are impressive. However, the existence of hospice provision is not a reason for excluding euthanasia as an option. The best testimony to the success of the hospice movement would be the euthanasia option's being available but being never taken up. In short, as long as economic circumstances and government spending policies make hospice care unavailable to many who would benefit from it, considerations of beneficence would indicate that euthanasia should be an available option. And, were hospice care to become a real option for all, considerations of autonomy would still support the availability of the euthanasia option. The two key questions are: Would continuing restrictions on autonomy really make hospice care generally available? And would the moral cost of restricting autonomy be worth the moral gain in terms of one view of good dying?

10.14 THE MORALITY OF NONVOLUNTARY EUTHANASIA

As we have seen, nonvoluntary euthanasia occurs when an individual is killed because it is believed to be in his best interests to die even though he cannot express any opinion on the decision. Can nonvoluntary euthanasia be morally justified? To facilitate our discussion we shall examine, first of all, the case of young infants and, second, the case of those who were once able to express a view on euthanasia but due to their present condition are not now.

(A) Nonvoluntary euthanasia: infanticide

In discussing infanticide, Glover (1977, p. 154) highlighted the following problem:

> Future medical advances, combined with a determination to save the lives of all foetuses, could lead to a greatly increased proportion of severely handicapped people in the population. As a result of current medical knowledge, sometimes combined with a determination to keep babies alive wherever possible, we are already moving in that direction. We are able to save premature babies at increasingly early stages of pregnancy, and as a result we save a higher proportion of people with severe defects. Operations on abnormal babies, and protection against what would otherwise be fatal illnesses, have the same result. Many more mentally subnormal babies survive; many more also survive with such handicaps as spina bifida.
>
> Only those with the crudest and most complacent outlook could feel that no problem exists. They easily accept either a blanket policy of infanticide or the misery caused by a policy of saving lives wherever possible. But for those who agree that there is a problem, it is often hard to know how to start thinking about it.

One recently expressed and immediate reaction to this line of thought is to accuse the author of harbouring a prejudice against handicapped individuals and voicing 'handicapism'. Handicapism is taken to represent an unwarranted bias or prejudice against individuals merely on account of the fact that they are handicapped. This prejudice is thought to be every bit as wrong as sexism or racism. Why should being handicapped pose any more problems than being male or Caucasian does?

One response to this question is to note that in cases of sex or race, whatever differences do exist are of no moral importance and do not justify treating different people differently; there are simply individuals who are male, female, Caucasian, Chinese, Negro, etc. and it is arbitrary and for that reason wrong to discriminate between them on the grounds of their sex or race. Indeed, many of the allegedly important differences have their real basis in cultural or social attitudes. On the other hand, it is claimed that handicapped individuals do suffer from real disadvantages which can be a ground for according them special treatment. However, whether the disadvantage is such that euthanasia may be thought required would depend not on the mere presence of the disadvantage but on whether the disability is so severe as to make the life not worth living.

Two kinds of consideration that can bear upon the rightness or wrongness of ending a life are considerations of autonomy and considerations
of the kind of life a person has or will have. From the perspective of
autonomy, whether or not an infant is handicapped is of no direct import.
This is so because young infants *per se* are not rational, self-conscious
persons; they are not autonomous individuals and, to that extent, as we
saw in the case of foetuses (see section 8.9, above), killing young infants
is not the same as killing mature adult persons. Infants, like foetuses, lack
the characteristics which normally make killing adult persons wrong. And
this point applies to all infants and not merely handicapped ones. From
the perspective of the future life they will enjoy or suffer, however, the
extent of hardship is morally relevant because normally the lives of young
infants are considered precious and thought worth preserving and cherish-
ing and it is only if, for example, there is believed to be the real probability
of leading a future wretched life that consideration would be given to the
possibility of allowing the infant to die. So, if handicapped infants are
ever justifiably killed, it is not because they have any less autonomy-based
right to life than 'normal' infants but must rather be for other reasons.

For ending the life of a handicapped infant to be an act of nonvoluntary
euthanasia, it must be believed that death would be in the infant's
interests; given its present condition or status and its possible future
existence, death is preferable to continuing to live and develop. Let us
see how it might be determined whether nonvoluntary euthanasia would
be appropriate, bearing in mind that nonvoluntary euthanasia involves a
judgement that for a certain infant, given its condition, death is preferable
to continuing to live.

Consider the case of Down's syndrome infants. There has been a
number of well-reported cases in the press involving the death of such
infants. Down's syndrome is a congenital defect affecting both the physical
and the mental development of the infant. Such infants have 47 chromoso-
mes instead of the normal 46 and have a distinctive physical appearance
as well as suffering mild to severe mental retardation. Is the future for
these infants such that nonvoluntary euthanasia is justified?

Kuhse and Singer (1985, p. 141) in commenting on Down's syndrome
infants state:

> Down's syndrome is especially problematic, because it is often possible
> for a Down's syndrome infant to live a reasonably happy, if simple, sort
> of life. An English judge of the Court of Appeal was swayed by this
> consideration in the case of a baby known to the public only as Alexan-
> dra. Alexandra was born in July 1981, in the London borough of
> Hammersmith. . . . she was a Down's syndrome infant with a life-
> threatening. blockage which needed surgical removal. The parents

refused consent for surgery. The Director of Hammersmith Social Services took the issue to court, where it was decided to make the child a ward of the court and to authorize the operation.

Following the court order, the infant was taken to a London hospital for surgery – where the surgeon refused to operate when he learned that the parents had refused consent. Another court hearing was called and this time the parents' decision was upheld. The case was finally decided on appeal. Lord Justice Templeman held that surgery should be performed, on the grounds that the life of a Down's syndrome infant is not 'demonstrably awful'. The decision implied that if the infant had had some other defect, with a 'demonstrably awful' life in store, surgery would not have been ordered.

It would seem that one would have to concur with the judge's judgement that the projected life of a Down's syndrome infant is not such that death would be preferable to life. But perhaps more can be said about such cases which might change this initial judgement. Kuhse and Singer (1985, p. 143) seem to believe this may be the case when they state the following in discussion of another case involving a rather more complicated operation:

> Down's syndrome is surely relevant to the decision to operate because it means a reduced potential for a life with the unique features which are commonly and reasonably regarded as giving special value to human lives. Even allowing for the more optimistic assessments of the potential of Down's syndrome children, this potential cannot be said to equal that of a normal child.

This is undoubtedly true; Down's syndrome children do not have the potential of a normal child. But where euthanasia is treated as an option the question is not whether the child's life will be worse than other people's but whether it will be worse than being dead. If Down's syndrome children *per se* were to be killed, could such killings be correctly described as euthanasic killings? Surely not, because euthanasic killings occur only when death, as opposed to continued life, is a benefit. And it is not demonstrably clear that this is true in the case of Down's syndrome children. The killing of an individual might be envisaged because of a perceived lower quality of life and/or the possible hardships this may impose on others, or indeed because of basically eugenic considerations. This has to be firmly distinguished from killing an individual for genuinely euthanasic reasons where given his present and projected condition death is identified as a clear benefit to him. (See the Linacre (1982) discussion on this p. 10; and Hursthouse, 1987, pp. xi–xii.)

Thus, if a Down's syndrome infant is killed, and there are no other complications which would materially and detrimentally affect the projected quality of life, this is not an instance of nonvoluntary euthanasia. However, such complications can exist and the prognosis can be such that death is perceived as a clear benefit. In such cases, the killing of such an infant would be an instance of nonvoluntary euthanasia; and the same consideration would apply to other defective infants. Where the foreseen and predicted future life of the infant is such that death is perceived as a benefit to it, then, and only then is the killing the infant an act of nonvoluntary euthanasia.

It is hard to identify a moral reason why nonvoluntary euthanasia should not take place on young infants whose life has every prospect of continuing to be one of pain and misery. There is one consideration that might be thought to count against killing infants: it is sometimes maintained that no one can be in a position to make judgements about the quality of someone else's life. We consider this in the next section.

(B) Nonvoluntary euthanasia: adult human beings

When nonvoluntary euthanasia is discussed in connection with adults, the kind of case considered is one in which an individual is no longer competent to express an opinion on his condition or on the worthwhileness of a proposed course of treatment. For example, he may have suffered permanent brain damage, or be in a coma. The health care team may be uncertain as to what treatment to offer. Given the condition and the predicted outcome of any treatment, some may advocate euthanasia, while others may refrain from such a judgement on the grounds that they are in no position to impose quality of life judgements as a basis for treatment or nontreatment. What guidelines can be offered?

First of all, the individual may have given some advice or instruction as to what would be appropriate treatment in such circumstances. This could be in the form of informal instructions to relatives or it could be more formal and written down in what is now referred to as a 'living will', a kind of advance directive for health care. In a living will, a person directs what specific treatments or measures ought to be employed or excluded, if at some later stage of his life he is incapable of making such decisions and requires care. In such circumstances, the existence of a living will and the instructions it contains may, if the advice is not to treat in specified circumstances, amount in fact to a request for voluntary euthanasia. Through the living will the person has spoken. What we have advocated earlier about voluntary euthanasia would apply here, given the need to respect individual autonomy. In consideration of such cases, the Linacre report (1982, p. 51) states:

there will be some who made a considered choice, while competent, about the medical care to be given or not given them during any later period of incompetence. If a doctor reasonably judges that that earlier considered choice has not been superseded by the passage of time, or by later indications of the patient's real wishes, or by substantial changes in the character of the treatment, he may reasonably consider himself entitled not to impose on that patient treatment thus rejected in advance, even if it may perhaps have been immorally rejected. The reason for this is that this patient's choice may here be considered to have the same force as the considered choice of a still competent patient, which even when it is apparently a choice for suicide by omission should not be overridden, since the patient's liberty and autonomy ought to be respected.

If no such advice is to hand, is it not appropriate, indeed necessary, to engage in quality of life judgements in determining whether to treat or not? Are they not unavoidable? On this point, the Linacre report (1982, p. 30) had the following to say:

> We do not deny that judgements which can (but need not) be called 'quality of life' judgements do enter into the process of medical decision-making. Any therapeutic recommendation is based on a consideration of likely and possible advantages and disadvantages that may accrue to the patient. The doctor makes some sort of comparison – weighing is too simple a metaphor – between the benefits and the risks and burdens for the patient that will or may accrue from the specific treatment under consideration. And this comparison is inevitably made against the background of the patient's present and likely condition and prognosis. So the questions being asked, implicitly, can be put thus: given his present 'quality of life', are the burdens of this (expensive or time-consuming or painful or disfiguring or undignified . . .) medical treatment worth enduring, in view of (a) the probable 'quality of his life' while undergoing it and (b) the probable 'quality of his life' if and when the treatment is completed.

However, for Linacre (1982), while such questions can and must be asked, the *reason* for asking them is important, because this will serve to distinguish the legitimate medical question from what Linacre (1982) views as the illegitimate euthanasic question.

> it is sufficient to notice the precise role of the question in trains of practical reasoning that are non-suicidal and non-euthanasiast: it focuses, and must be kept focused, on the advantages and disadvantages of specific possible treatments, given their effects, side-effects and out-

come. It does not enquire about, let alone focus upon, the worthwhile-ness of the patient's being alive at all.

The decision resulting from the non-euthanasiast practical reflection may be that no possible specific treatment is now, for this patient, worthwhile. And that decision may be arrived at in the knowledge that, untreated, the patient will probably die somewhat earlier than he would if treated. And indeed that consequence of the decision may be accepted without regret, and with the feeling, expressed or unexpressed, that death will bring relief to that patient. Still, such a decision can be perfectly reasonable and morally proper. But it would be euthanasiast, and so morally improper, if it used the judgement that death would bring relief, or that the patient's life was no longer worth living, or that the patient's prospective quality of life was too poor, as the basis for a decision to regard death as the objective, or an objective, of the treat-ments to be decided on.

(Linacre, 1982, pp. 30–31)

For Linacre (1982, p. 32) what is at issue here is the very objective of the caring mission.

The character of medical practice would be very radically altered, too, if quality of life judgements became a focus of practical reflection, rather than merely part of the background to the selection of appropriate treatment. For then opinions such as 'I'm glad his sufferings are over' or 'I hope death comes quickly to relieve him' would cease to be merely the comments of someone drawing attention to the miseries from which death would bring relief. Rather, such opinions would form the basis and criterion for selection of treatment, and the proper goals of treat-ment would be taken to include not only life, health and comfort, but also death itself. In the context of medical practice thus conceived, 'quality of life' opinions would function as practical judgements calling for death-dealing treatment.

Can the distinction Linacre 1982 is drawing here be sustained? Ought quality of life judgements only to be concerned with the selection of appropriate treatments, with appropriate means, and not with decisions as to whether death would be an appropriate end? Can, indeed, the two kinds of decision be separated ultimately?

As we have seen, in deciding not to treat one may be embracing the possibility that this decision will hasten death and this may be accepted with total equanimity if not relief. Can the hastening of the death be separated from the prior decision not to treat?

It would appear that Linacre 1982 is relying here on the 'double-effect' doctrine which claims that, while it may be acceptable to perform a right act even if you know that unsought and undesired consequences will result, it is never acceptable to perform a wrong act because you know acceptable and good consequences will follow. Thus, not to treat for acceptable medical reasons is morally permissible, even though an earlier death will be a predictable and not unwelcome consequence; but if the death of the patient is actively sought because it is believed to be in her best interests, it would be wrong to act with this as the objective of the nontreatment even though the consequences – the early death of the patient – would not be unacceptable and might be welcomed.

But why should actively seeking the death of a patient where death is perceived as a benefit be viewed as a paradigm instance of a wrong or bad act? Are there clear and indisputable instances of acts that are *per se* good and bad, and is it manifestly obvious that an act of euthanasia would be an instance of an unacceptably bad act?

Is it possible to separate in this rigid fashion the description of an act from a description of the consequences which will follow? Is the acceptable act of nontreatment merely that and only based on perceived benefits, and is the predicted earlier death only a consequence? Normally the knowledge that nontreatment will lead to an earlier death is a sufficient reason for offering treatment, it is not usually dismissed as a mere consequence, unacceptable or otherwise. If prolongation of life is generally perceived as a benefit, why is it not here?

If death will bring relief, and that is welcomed, is the judgement not being made that the patient's life is not worth living? Any comprehensive judgement concerning whether to treat or not treat cannot be limited to a mere analysis of the advantages or otherwise of certain courses of treatment; it must concern itself with wider and more fundamental questions concerning the quality of life of the patient and in particular whether the patient's life is worth living. This is unavoidable.

What particularly alarms health care teams in making quality of life judgements is the possibility that values which are dear to them may intrude and result in a judgement which is appropriate for them but distorted from the patient's point of view. They may make the mistake of reaching a conclusion informed by their own personal values and not the patient's (see section 2.3 above). However, the very fact that a health care team is alert to the possibility of their personal values intruding will, of itself, probably provide the best defence against this happening. Furthermore, quality of life judgements are as likely to involve judgements of impersonal value as of personal value when consideration is being given to the appropriateness of nonvoluntary euthanasia in the cases that are likely to be considered.

In sum, comprehensive health care may require making decisions that for some patients, unable to express their views, death is the best thing that can happen and it ought to be brought about. The requirement that health care teams cherish their patients is not incompatible with the recognition that the best interests of some of those patients would be served by the arrival of their death.

10.15 THE MORALITY OF ACTIVE AND PASSIVE EUTHANASIA

Active euthanasia involves taking specific means, such as injecting with a lethal solution, to terminate a patient's life because it is believed that given his condition death is in his interests. Passive euthanasia involves withholding specific treatment or care in order to allow a patient to die because it is believed it is in the interests of the patient to do so. In the latter case, the patient may be in a terminal stage of a particular disease and thus, when treatment is withheld, dies as a result of his underlying condition. Alternatively, it may be that the condition of the patient is not life-threatening and, death when it occurs, comes about because normal sustenance has been withheld.

Some maintain that the withholding of treatment in specified circumstances, even when it is done because it is believed to be in the interests of the patient and death is foreseen, is not a euthanasic act. The reason for so thinking may be philosophical/religious as represented in the Linacre report 1982. Alternatively, it may be based on legal considerations as all forms of euthanasia, where death is sought as an end, are legally impermissible. This latter consideration is particularly influential with the medical profession. For others, the withholding of treatment or care can be an euthanasic act and is to be preferred over active euthanasia primarily because it does not infringe the general societal prohibition on *direct* killing.

What is common here (though not shared by Linacre 1982) is the belief that allowing someone to die is morally preferable to direct killing. The reason for this belief seems to be the following: as directly killing an individual is to harm him, much less harm is done if by inactivity (or indeed activity, for in certain cases allowing to die involves acting) one merely permits or arranges the circumstances within which an individual dies. To act to bring about a bad state of affairs is more evil than to omit to act and thus allow the same bad state of affairs to occur. Actions, here, are more culpable than omissions.

The reason for preferring allowing to die as opposed to killing appears to be based on an assumed difference between acts and omissions. The validity and true import of the acts/omissions distinction has been extensively and exhaustively questioned. We do not wish to enter that controversy now, other than to say that, in the last analysis, we are not confident that there is a clear distinction present: omissions are very often kinds of actions. Be that as it may, we now wish to examine the relevance of this distinction for our euthanasia discussion.

Omissions, it is claimed, are preferable to actions because if a harmful state of affairs occurs it is better to have merely allowed it to happen than to have acted to bring it about. Thus, if someone dies, it is better to have merely allowed this to happen than to have directly brought it about. And given that death is normally a state of affairs that is not welcomed, it is better to allow an individual to die than to kill him.

But now we have reached the heart of the matter. In euthanasic deaths, death is not perceived as a harm, an evil to be avoided. If it is, then euthanasic reasons for the death are absent. Rather, death is welcomed; it is seen to be in the interests of the individual who is to die.

So if in euthanasic deaths, death is welcome, what then becomes of the acts/omissions distinction and its purported relevance to the euthanasia debate? Perhaps, ironically, it is this: If omitting to act and merely allowing evil to occur is to be preferred to action to bring about the same effect where the effect is evil, then, where the effect is good and to be welcomed, acting to bring about the desired and good effect is to be preferred to merely allowing or permitting good to take place. Thus, an advocate of the importance of the acts/omissions distinction ought to support active, not passive, euthanasia. (See a discussion of this issue by H. Goldman, 1980.)

There will be circumstances where genuinely humanitarian considerations may demand active euthanasia, other circumstances where there is no great moral difference between active and passive euthanasia, and still other circumstances where passive euthanasia morally suffices. What must be combatted is a moral preference for passive euthanasia predicated on the acts/omissions distinction, because such a preference betrays a deep misunderstanding and misapprehension as to the very nature of genuinely euthanasic killing.

ELEVEN

Respecting life and measuring its quality

'Inherent in nursing is respect for life', says the International Council of Nurses Code for Nurses (reprinted in Beauchamp and Childress, 1983, pp. 332–333). There is sometimes a temptation to suppose that when respect for life is brought into play, considerations about the quality of life must be excluded. In this chapter we consider what respect for life involves and we explore what is and what is not involved in measuring the quality of life.

11.1 WHAT LIFE IS TO BE RESPECTED?

In some contexts, the word 'life' might refer to whatever distinguishes organic from inorganic matter. However, in the present context the point is not to mark off bacteria, seaweed, wasps, dogs and humans from lifeless rock. The life which is to be respected in nursing has to be more narrowly demarcated. *Roughly*, it is human life that is meant when we say that respect for life is inherent in nursing. But what is it *exactly?*

One possibility is that all human life and no other kind of life is to be respected. How might there be reason for this? A suggestion here is that there is something special that all humans have and nothing else has. A belief that is relevant to this line of thought is the belief that humans, and no other living creatures, have immortal souls. Thus possession of an immortal soul is the special thing that all humans have and nothing else has. Provided each human being receives a soul the instant it starts to live and ceases to have a soul the instant it ceases to live, this would give a reason for respecting all and only human life.

Many thinkers have seen difficulties with a view of this sort. The idea that there is a soul present from the moment of conception is a relatively recent one and is not accepted by all who believe in souls. Likewise, it is hard to be sure that a soul continues to be present in an ageing body as long as there is ventilation and a pulse. This may prompt questions about the status of a living human body before it receives a soul or after it has ceased to have one. Nevertheless, there are thinkers who consider it worth continuing the search for an understanding of the preciousness of human life along these lines.

Another idea is that each human life is to be respected because it is 'one of us', because all human beings are one another's kin. The suggestion here is that we ought to treat human beings in a different way from the way we treat any other creatures just because of their membership of the human species.

There is a well-known line of criticism of this suggestion which was noted in section 8.9 and which we now consider further. Peter Singer (1979, pp. 48–54) has argued that to ground special treatment solely on the basis of membership of a particular species is to display a form of prejudice or discrimination like racism or sexism. Species membership, just like mere membership of a particular race or sex, is a characteristic devoid of moral significance and is thus not an appropriate basis on which to ground special or privileged treatment. Granted that racism and sexism represent unjustifiable prejudices, speciesism, relying on the mere biological fact of membership of a species, must also be unacceptable. Thus mere membership of a species – *Homo sapiens* in the present case – is not a moral reason why a creature ought to be treated differently.

One response to Singer's 1979 argument may be expressed like this: 'But there is good reason to treat human beings differently from other living creatures; human beings have self-awareness, a rich and complex mental life, sophisticated desires and hopes, and the ability to form and elaborate and refine comprehensive and detailed plans.' The idea here is that, while unreasoned discrimination in favour of our own species would be comparable to unreasoned racial or sexual discrimination, there may be discrimination in favour of humans which is not unreasoned and therefore is importantly different from racism and sexism. We see lives which display self-consciousness and the associated mental characteristics as evoking respect and thus, from a moral point of view, as demanding the greatest protection. We can speak here of 'ultimate respect' to express the idea that the respect in question is not derivative or dependent on some further conditions being fulfilled over and above the possession of the characteristics just mentioned.

This response is entirely consistent with the conclusion of Singer's 1979 argument. Singer's 1979 conclusion is that mere species membership is not a good enough reason for according ultimate respect to a creature. The response just considered does not involve presenting *species member-*

ship as reason for ultimate respect; it rather offers other reasons – self-awareness, the ability to elaborate plans, etc. – for such respect.

Some philosophers have wanted to treat the characteristics listed as constituting personhood and have argued that persons should have ultimate respect, and that the level of respect accorded to other life-forms should depend on the level of consciousness present and the relative sophistication of their mental development. Be that as it may, we now have an indication of how to develop criteria to apply to different life-forms and species and to assess the level of respect they should have.

Whatever might be the truth about the meaning of the word 'person', the important thing is the presence in an individual of the characteristics we have mentioned as calling for ultimate respect and thus the reason why absolute protection is required. According to the current suggestion, it is the presence of these characteristics that makes life valuable. The use of the word 'person' to refer to this is convenient, but it can be dispensed with if it raises problems.

Rationality and the other characteristics associated with self-consciousness are typically found in human lives. But, should they be found to be present in nonhuman lives, then according to the present suggestion those lives too are to have the same respect. If there are angels and they have the characteristics in question then angelic life is to be respected. If future astronauts encounter life forms genetically unrelated to us but having those characteristics then they are to be respected as well. If further enquiry reveals dolphins or whales or chimpanzees to have those characteristics to a high degree then withholding such respect from them could not be justified.

In short, the present suggestion extends the boundaries of ultimate respect beyond the boundaries of our species. Whether we humans are alone within those boundaries or have nonhuman company, it is not our species membership which is the basis for ultimate respect of the kind of life we have; the basis for such respect is rather a set of characteristics which – at least in theory – we could turn out to have in common with members of other species.

There may be a case, as we have now seen, for extending the limits of ultimate respect so that they possibly encompass members of species other than our own. If this is correct then not *only* human life is to be respected. Another question is whether *all* members of our own species are to be within the limits. One suggestion here is that levels of respect for life are to be fixed a species at a time, so that the lives of all members of a species are due respect at not less than the level due to the lives of typical members of that species. Another suggestion is that it is as individuals and not as species members that we are due respect. If this is correct then the considerations noted above indicate not only that ultimate respect may be due to the lives of some nonhumans but also that it may not be due to the lives of all humans.

In pursuing this last suggestion one may seek to modify it by noting first that, in effect, normal mature humans merit ultimate respect in the first instance, and then proceeding to extend the scope of that respect to others (notably abnormal and infant humans). This extension may be attempted either by reference to some relation holding between normal adults and other humans or by reference to the idea that the others are on the way to becoming mature adults or are unlike normal mature adults only by misfortune (cf. Holland, 1984).

Another approach involves focusing on a biographical rather than bio-logical understanding of the word 'life'. When we say that someone has an interesting life or that their life is full of disappointments we are not making reference to biological facts (see Rachels, 1986, p. 25). A life has the features of a story. The things that a person does and that befall her in her life have to be understood in the context of that narrative. Here the focus is not on whether a living being has certain psychological attributes at a given point in time but rather on whether that being is living a narrative that unfolds over a period of time.

In this section we have sought to show that there are several distinct lines of thought concerning the preciousness of life to be explored. Philos-ophers are continuing to work at exploring them.

11.2 WHAT IS INVOLVED IN RESPECTING LIFE?

At the very least, to respect life of a certain kind is to regard the fact that an action will save a life of that kind as a reason for taking that action, and to regard the fact that a certain action will involve loss of life of that kind as a reason for not taking that action. In other words, to respect life of a certain kind is to treat a being with life of that kind as having moral standing.

At the upper limit, respecting life of a certain kind is treating the fact that an action will cost life as a supremely decisive reason for not taking that action; it is to take the view that no reason could ever be a good enough reason to justify taking a life of that kind. Such respect is some-times expressed as a sanctity of life principle. Once this principle is selected and applied at stage 3 of deliberation, it generates stage 4 considerations which override all other stage 4 considerations in decisively ruling out certain courses of action. We saw this in discussing how such a principle would operate in connection with abortion and euthanasia. This does not mean that considerations of quality of life can play no role with regard to other options. They are overruled when they might have counted in favour of a course of action which respect for life rules out. But they remain relevant to the choice of other courses of action. Thus rejecting euthanasia on sanctity of life grounds is consistent with favouring hospice care on quality of life grounds.

Respecting human life in this way amounts to embracing a judgement of impersonal value whereby human life is judged to have value of a special kind. What is special about it is that, as a practical stage 4 consideration, it outweighs all other considerations of value, no matter how weighty they are. And, in as much as the judgement is of impersonal value, it is to the effect that the value is not relative to priorities and ways of living a life that might vary from one person to another. Given this judgement it is appropriate to rule out euthanasia as an option even in the case where the person whose life it is wants to die. As we saw, in sections 10.4 and 10.5, one would have to have very powerful reasons for taking this position, and it is hard to see how anyone could see themselves as entitled to take it except possibly within a religious framework.

One way of respecting life is attributing to human life an impersonal value that overrides all other value, rights, and other considerations. Respecting life might also mean attributing to it value without that power to override. Or it might mean acknowledging a right to life. It might even mean a bit of each.

Not respecting life is regarding it as not counting for anything at all. For example, when insects killed by hitting the car windscreen are regarded as nothing but a nuisance, their insect life is not respected. Embryonic human life may be not respected. Or it may be accorded a lower degree of respect than conscious personal life by being treated as counting for less than conscious personal life. (This would be the case if, other things being equal, a court awarded a smaller sum of money in compensation for the death of an embryo than for the death of a salesperson.) One quite common view is that human life before birth has value and that the value increases – becomes more weighty as a stage 4 consideration – as it develops. On this view abortion may need justifying, as there is *some* reason for not taking a foetus's life, and early abortion does not need much justification while more and more powerful justificatory reasons are needed as time goes on and the foetus develops. Having moral standing could here be thought of as having a life that counts for something, a life which others have some reason not to take. One might think moral standing or the value of human life is small at conception and gradually moves along a continuum of greater standing or value. Or one might think of it as zero at conception and as becoming positive at some later point and gradually increasing from then.

A different idea is the idea of respecting life as respecting a right. Here the idea is that people have lives to live. According to the autonomy principle, a person's conception of how to live and their plans for living their life are to be respected. A person's autonomy is violated when their plans for their own life are set aside and subjected to someone else's plans. An especially deep and serious way of violating someone's plans for their life is to take their life, thereby putting an end to all their plans. According to the principle of autonomy such violation is wrong; it is a wrong of the worst kind.

In discussing the kind of sanctity of life principle which requires life to be preserved even against the interests and wishes of the person whose life it is, we found it hard to identify secular grounds for such a principle. However, a secular principle of respect for life can be held every bit as firmly, sincerely, and intensely as a religious principle of the sanctity of life. Suppose involuntary euthanasia or nonresuscitation were to be proposed in the case of a patient whose life is plainly no longer worth living but who stubbornly insists that they want to be resuscitated when the inevitable next arrest comes. Someone who finds autonomy-based considerations among the most powerful of stage 4 considerations will be at least as firm in resisting the proposal for euthanasia or nonresuscitation as an adherent of the sanctity of life. So an autonomy-based respect for life should not be thought of as softer than adherence to the sanctity of life. The difference is one of scope rather than one of strength. An autonomy-based respect for life recognizes a right to life making it as wrong as anything can be to take a person's life against that person's will; but it also admits a right that a person has to lay aside their own life or to waive their right to life. It thus differs from an insistence on a sanctity of life which makes it as wrong as anything can be to take a person's life regardless of what the person wants. In short, from a sanctity of life point of view, whether a person wants to live or not counts for nothing; from an autonomy-based respect for life point of view, the will of the person whose life it is counts for everything.

Having reviewed some things that respect for life might mean and how considerations of respect for life can feature at stage 4 of deliberation, let us finally note that there is nothing about such considerations that invalidates considerations of the quality of life. Respecting life and upholding the sanctity of life are perfectly consistent with believing some lives to be better than others. Respect for life does not imply that there can be no judging the quality of a person's life. What may be insisted on, however, is that the sanctity of life or an autonomy-based right to life can be a decisive consideration counting against a course of action and overriding all considerations of quality that might otherwise have counted for that action.

So respect for life does not make considerations of the quality of life unintelligible or illegitimate. We now turn to consider what is involved in judgements of quality of life and how quality might be measured.

11.3 GOOD LIVES AND POOR ONES

If we learn something about the conditions of human life at a place and time remote from our own, we often have little difficulty in coming to have a view about whether people's life there and then was better or worse than ours. We should be a bit cautious in taking such a view. We should not too hastily dismiss the possibility that more information about those conditions of life or greater imaginative understanding of them would change our value judgement. But granted a fair share of information and imagination, there does not seem to be any problem about judging life under some circumstances to be better than life under other circumstances.

It is surely in order to look back over a century, or a decade, or a year, and to wonder whether human life is now better or worse than it used to be, or to wonder whether life for some groups of people is now better or worse than it used to be. We might speculate about whether a typical child's life in Britain now is better or worse than a generation ago. We might speculate about whether life will be better or worse in the middle of the next century.

Often, when someone has died, we thank goodness their suffering is over; on other occasions we think it would have been better if the deceased person had lived longer. When we thank goodness, it is often because we think the life they were living was a wretched life and not a good life; often, though, we think the death is a great shame, and we think this in part because we think the life the person was having was a good life. Among all the quirky things that are perhaps present in our hopes about the kinds of lives our children and grandchildren will have, there are also some uncontroversial things. For example, if we want our children to be healthy, wealthy and wise, we are wishing them what most people would acknowledge to be (at least provided the wealth is not excessive) a good life.

In short, judging some lives to be better than others, judging life under some circumstances to be better than life under other circumstances, judging some parts of a person's life to be better than other parts of that person's life – making such judgements is a quite normal activity. We may disagree, sometimes, with one another's judgements; but we seldom query the whole idea of thinking that life can vary in quality.

Intellectual humility is in order. A person who takes a pitying or contemptuous view of the quality of a nun's life, or a rugby player's, or a librarian's, or an uneducated person's may come to an unsound assessment of quality for want of imagination or appreciation; the judgement may reflect a loutish incomprehension of spiritual joys, an over-genteel lack of insight into the exhilaration of rough and tumble, a coarse ignorance of literary culture, or a blinkered disdain for any other culture. Those who

take the view that the life that a severely handicapped baby is likely to have is a wretched life are sometimes accused of insensitivity and arrogance. In supposing a life to be good or poor we do need to be on our guard against such moral and intellectual defects in ourselves. Still, with due caution we need not despair of arriving at sound, reasonable views about how a life or part of a life may be better or worse than another.

11.4 QUANTIFYING THE QUALITY OF LIFE

As noted in section 11.3, there is nothing strange or unfamiliar about having views on the quality of a life. At the very least we can make some rough comparisons. But it might be thought that only severely limited knowledge of this kind is to be had. Perhaps such knowledge is unavoidably vague. Perhaps it is especially fragile because if I make such a judgement (e.g. that a friend who is living in Italy has a better life than a friend who has gone to live in the United States) and someone who has the same information as I do questions it, there is no reason I can give them in support of my judgement; all I can do is invite them to think again. And perhaps there is too much incommensurability for comfort; no doubt a long and joyful life is better than a short and dull one, but can a longer dull life be compared with a shorter joyful one? There are various ways in which life can be better or worse; if Amelia's life is better than Brenda's in some of those ways and worse than it in others, which of them has the better life overall? If only a life like Amelia's and a life like Brenda's are on offer, which one am I to hope for for my child?

To consolidate judgements of the value of different lives it would be useful to be able to take different factors which are known to make a life better or worse, and to know *how much* difference each factor makes. Exceptions aside, having eye teeth is better than not having eye teeth; and being able to play the guitar is better than not being able to play the guitar. If we knew *how much* worse life without eye teeth is than life with eye teeth and we knew *how much* better life with the ability to play the guitar is than life without the ability to play the guitar, then we could know whether losing one's eye teeth and acquiring the ability to play the guitar leaves one better or worse off. To the extent that the difference between having eye teeth and not having them can be compared with the difference between being able to play the guitar and not being able to play it, we can speak of a *trade-off* between factors – and speak of a change for the worse being (partially or fully) compensated for by a different change for the better. Granted that life has got in some ways better in the last fifty years and in some ways worse, if we can say how much each of those ways makes life better or worse then we can perhaps work out whether life is now better or worse overall. And, granted some intelligent guesses about ways in which lives would have been better and worse if things had been otherwise (e.g. if the National Health Service had not been founded, or if the Russian Revolution had not occurred), if we can say how much each of those ways makes people's lives better or worse, we can perhaps say whether people's lives are better or worse lives overall than they would otherwise have been.

It would be extremely ambitious to seek to quantify the difference that every change in quality makes to life. The magnitude of the task is overwhelming. A more limited objective would be to focus on health-related ways in which life can be better or worse and to find out how much difference each of those makes to the quality of life. Some progress has been made towards this objective.

We can say how much difference the presence of a quality makes if we can correlate the difference between the presence and the absence of the quality with the difference between amounts of some quantity. One such quantity has been extensively considered, namely duration. Suppose, for example, it was found that having ten years of life with only one leg was just about as good as having seven years of (otherwise similar) life with two legs; then the qualitative difference between having both of one's legs and only having one of them would be correlated with the quantitative difference between ten and seven. Suppose also that it was found that having ten years of life with no taste was just as good as having six and a half otherwise similar years of life with the ability to taste one's food. Then it could be shown that, other things being equal, losing the power of taste is worse than losing a leg.

11.5 VALUE ENQUIRY – PREFERENCES AS EVIDENCE

How might such correlations be established? For a start one can compare pairs of possibilities oneself. Think about ten years of life with no significant discomfort and about thirteen years of life with constant low-level pain, and judge which is better. (For the purpose of trying this out, the reader may choose a low-level pain that they recently experienced; or, if remembering it is hard, wait until life brings another one and then ponder whether ten years without it would or would not be better than thirteen years with it.) Thinking about the two possibilities and judging which is better is a bit like inspecting two scarves and judging which is more yellow in colour.

Choose a certain level of pain and see whether you can make the comparison. Then try it with a different level of pain. See if there is a level of pain so low that, in your judgement, getting an extra three years of life at the cost of enduring that pain would plainly be worth it. Then see if there is a level of pain severe enough to make the gain in time plainly not worth having. In between will be a region where you hesitate. Locating that region amounts to finding out your current (no doubt inexact) views about the relative values of pain and duration.

This kind of comparison is all right as far as it goes, but the person doing the comparing might be unusual in some way, or might simply be mistaken. So it is reasonable to seek corroboration by getting other opinions; it is reasonable to ask a lot of different people to compare the same two possibilities and judge which is better; and it is reasonable to include people with personal experience of the possibilities being considered. If everyone turns out to agree with the initial judgement then there is no reason to suppose that that judgement was incorrect. If almost everyone disagrees with the initial judgement then there is reason to suppose the initial agreement was incorrect. If significant numbers of different people make conflicting judgements then there is reason to suspect that the question is just a matter of opinion and that there is, so to speak, no fact of the matter.

Thus a way to get evidence as to which of two possibilities is better is to ask a lot of people to think about the two possibilities and judge which is better. If virtually everyone comes up with the same answer then that is the answer you were after.

The procedure just envisaged is pretty rough and ready. Alan Williams has described something more refined. First, one needs to identity some factors that affect quality of life. Kind *et al.* (1982) have identified two such factors – disability and distress – and have further identified eight degrees of disability and four degrees of distress, listed in Table 11.5.

Table 11.5 Disability and distress factors

Distress	A. No distress
	B. Mild
	C. Moderate
	D. Severe
Disability	1. No disability
	2. Slight social disability
	3. Severe social disability and/or slight impairment of performance at work, able to do all housework except very heavy tasks
	4. Choice of work or performance at work very severely limited, housewives and old people able to do light housework only but able to go out shopping
	5. Unable to undertake any paid employment, unable to continue any education, old people confined to home except for escorted outings and short walks and unable to do shopping,

housewives able only to perform a few simple tasks
6. Confined to chair or to wheelchair or able to move around in the house only with support from an assistant
7. Confined to bed
8. Unconscious.

Disability state 1 can coexist with each of the four distress states; so we can distinguish four states that a person might be in – 1A, 1B, 1C, and 1D. Disability state 2 can likewise coexist with each of the four distress states, so again there are four different states that a person with that degree of disability might be in. The same goes for the third degree of disability, and for each of the others except for unconsciousness. Counting them up we find that twenty nine distinct states that a person might be in have been identified.

A person can be shown a list of these states and asked to judge how bad each state is.

If the healthy state is said to be equal to 1, and dead is equal to 0, then respondents can then be asked to attach a number (less than 1) to each of the other states. . . . Thus a state valued at 0.5 is felt to be only half the value as being healthy would be, with the implication that two years life expectancy in that state is felt to be of equal value to one year of healthy life expectancy.

(Williams, 1985a, p. 4)

It is not clear that Williams 1985a regards conclusions obtained from data of this kind as conclusions about impersonal value. (He says that 'in a democracy no one can really set themselves up as experts in what other people's values ought to be' (pp. 4–5), which suggests that he has in mind personal rather than impersonal values.) However, they can be so regarded. Just as our conclusions about our personal values have to be tentative, for we cannot rule out the possibility that – like Midas – we have more to learn about what is important to us personally, so also conclusions about impersonal values have to be tentative and provisional, subject to corroboration or change at a later date. A respondent may, with more experience, come to reverse their comparative valuation of two states; their responses may have been distorted by insufficient information or by insufficient imagination to appreciate what it would be like to be in a certain state. The convergent value judgements of a lot of people are the best evidence we could have for quantitative conclusions about the effect of distress and disability factors on a person's quality of life. If a better way than this of establishing judgements of impersonal value can be devised, then the improved way should replace the existing way. In the absence of a better way, it seems reasonable to proceed with this way, always bearing in mind that our best-corroborated conclusions are still tentative in character.

11.6 WHAT ARE QALYS?

A QALY is a Quality Adjusted Life Year. Two benefits of health care are the prolongation of life and the improvement of life. By promoting these, health care activities are supposed to do good. But they are distinct; consequently efforts directed at one of them will not necessarily always promote the other. To be reasonably sure that efforts can be directed where they will do most good, it would be very useful to relate prolongation and improvement in such a way that it would be possible to tell when more good can be done by improvement and when more good can be done by prolongation. Then prolonging life and improving life could be brought under one heading instead of two separate ones. This is what QALYs are intended to make possible. Benefits gained in the form of prolongation of life and benefits gained in the improvement of life could both be seen – and measured – as gains in QALYs.

Suppose it is known how many years of life can be expected to be gained as a result of certain health care intervention. This is an expected gain in terms of the prolongation of life. To find out the gain in terms of the prolongation-cum-improvement, one has to make adjustments to take account of the quality of life. Adjustments can be made with the aid of **quality adjustment factors**. If a certain state of health can be taken to be only half as good as full health, then the relevant quality adjustment factor is 0.5; six unadjusted years of life in that state could then be deemed equivalent to three quality adjusted life years (i.e. 6×0.5 QALYs).

In general, life years can be converted to QALYs, given the health states in which those years are lived, provided appropriate adjustment factors are to hand. There are different methods of arriving at adjustment factors (Loomes and McKenzie, 1989; McCulloch, 1990) and comparative work on them continues. One approach is that of Kind *et al.* (1982) outlined in section 11.5, above. The adjustment factors arrived at on the basis of interviews with 70 subjects are as follows:

Table 11.6 Quality adjustment factors, based on subject interviews (Kind *et al.*, 1982), used to calculate QALYs

		DISTRESS			
		A	B	C	D
	1	1.000	0.995	0.990	0.967
	2	0.990	0.986	0.973	0.932
DISABILITY	3	0.980	0.972	0.956	0.912
	4	0.964	0.956	0.942	0.870

Table 11.6 contd.

5	0.946	0.935	0.900	0.700
6	0.875	0.845	0.680	0.000
7	0.677	0.564	0.000	−1.486
8	−1.028	–	–	–

(There are no states 8B, 8C or 8D as unconsciousness precludes distress states B, C, and D.)

With this matrix, a number of life years in a given state of disability and distress can be multiplied by the quality adjustment factor for that state to yield a number of QALYs.

11.7 QALYS AND PRACTICE

It is often argued in the United Kingdom that the amount of public money allocated to the health service should not be significantly increased because the demand for health care is limitless. This is not a good argument. Good arguments would have to show that significantly increasing health service expenditure would take money away from more important things, or that taxpayers are not willing to support increased health service expenditure, or that increased health service expenditure would discourage private initiatives, or that the same benefits can be obtained more efficiently in another way.

Be that as it may, there is reason to think that, even if health service expenditure was considerably increased, there would still be insufficient resources to meet all health care needs. This is partly because some health care activity is life-saving. If a person's need for life-saving treatment is unfulfilled that person subsequently has no further needs; but if a person's need for life-saving treatment is fulfilled then, in many cases, the person will subsequently have further needs. Also, technical developments often make it possible to fulfil needs which could not be fulfilled previously; they thus introduce scope for additional expense (cf. Gillon, 1989).

So the problem of how to decide which health care needs are to be met and which are not is not a problem we could easily spend our way out of. With available resources there are a great many health care needs each of which we could choose to meet, but only by choosing not to meet some of the others. Decisions have to be made about priorities, so that resources can be targeted on activities with high priority; and there has to be efficiency, so that more health benefits rather than less are achieved from the expenditure that is made.

Given quantitative conclusions about the differences between different states of health that a person might be in, and given information about treatments which alter people's state of health, we can quantify the health benefits produced by those treatments. Where a health care activity prolongs life, the years of life gained are (usually) a benefit. And whether or not a treatment is life-saving, by taking account of the quality of life brought about by the treatment we can in principle quantify the benefits brought about by the treatment.

> The essence of a QALY is that it takes a year of healthy life expectancy to be worth 1, but regards a year of unhealthy life expectancy as worth less than 1. Its precise value is lower the worse the quality of life of the unhealthy person (which is what the 'quality adjusted' bit is all about). If being dead is worth zero, it is, in principle, possible for a QALY to be negative, i.e. for the quality of someone's life to be judged as worse than being dead.
>
> The general idea is that a beneficial health care activity is one that generates a positive amount of QALYs, and that an efficient health care activity is one where the cost-per-QALY is as low as it can be. A high priority health care activity is one where the cost-per-QALY is low, and a low priority activity is one where cost-per-QALY is high.
>
> (Williams, 1985a, p. 3)

A small example of the kind of comparison thus permitted:

> A treatment which offered the prospect of four years of healthy life expectancy in place of four years in a state valued at 0.75, would be 'worth' 1 QALY (0.25 of a QALY is gained each year for four years), whereas a treatment which moved someone from a state valued at 0.25 to one valued at 0.75 for four years would be worth two QALYs.
>
> (Williams, 1985a, p. 4)

11.8 AN INELIMINABLE MORAL FRICTION

Even if two states of affairs are very dreadful ones, it may be possible to judge that one is less bad than the other. But we should not be too quick to assume that producing either of them would be right, even for an agent who had no other option. G. E. M. Anscombe has said

> . . . if someone really thinks, *in advance*, that it is open to question whether such an action as procuring the judicial execution of the innocent should be quite excluded from consideration – I do not want to argue with him; he shows a corrupt mind.
>
> (Anscombe, 1981, p. 40)

What might the corruption consist in? It might consist in being ready to take it that one of the available options is right when each of them is known to be wrong. Suppose someone asks what a person in such a situation is supposed to do. The answer that they had better minimize the harm produced is a plausible one. But it is perhaps also plausible to say that each of the options is such that anyone taking them is soiled by it, and that where this is the case only a corrupted notion of *right* permits any course of action to be called right. Some situations are such that none of the available courses of action is right. Bernard Williams describes such a situation (Smart and Williams, 1973, pp. 98–99): a man is placed in a situation where 20 innocent people will be murdered unless he kills one of them; thus the two courses of action open to him are to kill one innocent person and to permit the killing of 20 innocent persons; and both of these options are wrong.

When we think of a case like this one, it is plausible to suppose that questions of right and wrong action are distinct from questions of value. For it is pretty plain that one outcome (one innocent person dead) is better – or less bad – than the other (20 innocent persons dead); and yet it is not at all plain that one course of action is right and the other not. So we can be clear about the answer to the question about the value of the outcomes and yet not be clear about the answer to the question of what is right; and if we can be clear about the answer to one understood question and unclear about the answer to another understood question, then they must be two different questions.

When one starts with the question of how best to use the available resources for health care, it is hard to see how anything other than seeking to achieve the best could be defended. When one starts with a consideration of individual patients one is bound to find it morally intolerable that a needy individual who could quite easily be made well should not get the treatment they need; and the moral intolerableness will be sensed all the more keenly by someone who is engaged in a caring relationship with the person in question. The two standpoints are both unavoidable and yet there is what Hollis calls 'an ineliminable moral friction' (Bell and Mendus, 1988, p. 18) between them.

The objective view of the agent who is responsible for matters of macroallocation and the participant view of the health professional facing individual patients or clients resist integration into a single coherent view. This resistance is perplexing. But Thomas Nagel (1986, p. 4) is perhaps right to say 'Certain forms of perplexity . . . seem to me to embody more insight than any of the supposed solutions to those problems.'

Recent discussion of QALYs has revealed or revived some problems that stubbornly resist satisfactory solution. One no-nonsense way of responding to problems that are plainly not going to be satisfactorily solved is to turn away from them. However the moral insights and concerns that underlie the most stubborn problems about resource allocation are too important for that. Simply turning away from them would be ceasing to care about things that we cannot decently give up caring about.

While health care has to be delivered in the way that will produce the best outcomes, the fact that (as John Harris's writings insist) this will involve wrongs means that there is an abiding moral unsatisfactoriness that has to be lived with.

11.9 QUALITY AND SCARCE RESOURCES

There are many detailed arguments for and against the application of a measure such as the quality adjusted life year. Significantly, the concluding comments of section 11.8 remind us of the inherent tension of having both an individual patient view and a sense of just distribution of health care resources. Perhaps we should decide at this point to agree with Nagel (1986) and begin to view the tension as useful in the sorts of additional insights it gives us rather than attempt to reach any satisfactory resolution of the conflict.

While this view might satisfy the more intellectual reader it will do nothing to meet the needs of the practitioner, particularly in the light of current health care reforms. Calculating QALYs, in one sense, is a rather esoteric way of making decisions about scarce health care resources. What has come in its wake is the much more radical introduction of an internal health market within the national health system.

From 1 April 1991, health authorities in England and Wales have become purchasers of health services from specialist hospital units and from community services. Each purchasing authority is allocated a sum of money related to the volume of service expected to meet the identified needs of the community which it serves. General practitioners are the key actors in such a scenario as they serve as the front line practitioners identifying illness and disease and determining which patients need more specialist treatment. Contracts between the providers of the services and the purchasers have been drawn up to determine how much is being offered, at what cost and at what quality.

Even with this very simplified explanation of the changes and before there is sufficient information to show whether it will be successful or not, a number of issues have emerged illustrating that the brave new world of the market place has done little to reduce the inevitable moral friction. For example, many professional groups have resisted the direct linkage of service provision with the day-to-day treatment of individual patients.

This argument has been illustrated in ways such as general practitioners resenting the fact that they may not be able to prescribe for their patients drugs which they believe they need because the doctor is overspent on his budget. Similarly a consultant physician argued that he would not wish to have to make the final decision of treating a middle aged man with lung cancer because the prognosis of such cases was very poor and, in financial terms not worth it. His argument was that it is much better for the practitioners to work to the principle of doing everything they can for the patients in front of them while someone else makes the resource decision. Conversely, an argument put forward by another consultant involved in transplant surgery suggested that a more judicious use of resources without the heroic attempts at treatment above all else would greatly increase the effectiveness of the service.

The need for each health authority to construct a detailed health profile of the community may be one secure point to start off a debate on matching need with resources. But as we saw with the QALY debate, how do you make a judgement between the need for treatment of ten kidney patients as opposed to 100 fractured hip cases if both groups were to take up the same amount of resources? One recent experiment carried out in the State of Oregon decided to ask the public to choose. Out of a list of dozens of treatments they were asked to prioritize the sorts of services they would be willing to support financially. Surprisingly – or not – the group chose to finance less expensive high technology treatments and supported more low key preventative health care programmes. For example, the respondents chose to support the antenatal care of 100 mothers rather than the care of premature babies with poor life expectancy. Whether this sort of experiment could be or should be replicated in the United Kingdom is an interesting question, particularly as it raises the question whether the choices made reflect personal values rather than judgements based on ethical principles. Would such a system reduce the dilemma of the individual practitioner who was still left to care for the particular patient?

Perhaps we are in danger of discussing the concepts of justice and fair allocation of resources rather than the notion of quality of life. Yet we can see that the arguments put forward earlier in this chapter apply equally to any mechanism used to ration resources. Broad guidelines are needed of course to help determine health policy and if such guidelines explicitly embrace notions such as equity, availability, accessibility and universality of service then the parameters exist for helping individual practitioners make good decisions about how they spend their resources. However, the existence of such guidelines does not diminish the potential moral conflict faced by a group of practitioners or an individual when it comes to making a judgement about what is best for another person.

While the quality of life debate can be and increasingly is construed in cost benefit analysis language, another perhaps more positive note to strike is to consider how existing resources can be used more effectively. This means that instead of attempting to ask the prior question of who should get what, we employ ourselves by considering whether we are using existing resources to the best effect for our clients. For example, a group of nurses on a care of the elderly ward decided to improve the quality of care they were providing to several elderly incontinent old ladies. They worked out that if they were to purchase a number of raised toilet seats for the existing facilities they would be able to bring the elderly residents to the toilet rather than allowing them to wet their undergarments. The initial reaction to the suggestion from the hospital manager was that they had no further resources for such equipment until the staff illustrated that the money saved in laundry costs would off-set the initial capital outlay in equipment.

Even this relatively straightforward example shows that unless a particular perspective in patient care is sensitive to quality of life issues then certain more negative ways of operating will creep in. It certainly was not in the patients' best interests to be incontinent and did not do a lot for their feeling of self-esteem. Until the group of nurses decided to try alternative ways of tackling the problem the quality of life for such patients was undeniably reduced.

This example offers a totally different view of the quality of life debate, namely what cumulative effect nurses and doctors have upon the overall experience of the patient. If we remove the resource argument even from this situation we are left with the question of how do nurses and doctors make judgements about the nature of the experience they are offering to their patients. Perhaps most professionals do not tend to see their discrete interventions in ways which either add to or detract from the overall life experience of the individual. Literature exploring the experience of chronic illness is replete with stories of how careless remarks made by professionals have had quite bad effects on patients. In such situations an element of mistrust creeps in and the patient tends not to believe that the effort is really in their best interests.

If this is – as is often stated – the case, then for professionals to talk about quality of life issues is rather false unless it is spoken about in impersonal resource-allocations ways. Again we are reminded of the inherent tension, the inevitable moral friction, of trying to ensure a quality of experience for one patient and perhaps by that very action denying another patient a similar experience. Can the professional reconcile the wider debates about resource allocation with the day-to-day experience of providing a quality service to enhance the patients' quality of life?

Studies such as McNeil *et al.* (1981) have indicated that professional and lay views of what constitutes a quality existence may be at odds. It may be that given the choice the middle aged man with lung cancer does not wish for heroic attempts at treatment. It may also be that elderly ladies do not mind sitting in wet undergarments. Perhaps as potential judges or arbitrators of such situations it is incumbent upon us as nurses and doctors to at least know the answers to these sorts of questions.

TWELVE

Caring in nursing – do we need to bother?

In a recent play by Alan Bennett (1988) called *A Cream Cracker under the Settee*, we are party to the deliberations of a character called Doris. Unfortunately, Doris, who is in her seventies, fell when she was trying to dust a cupboard top and has fractured her hip. We hear how, stranded in her semidetached living room, she reaches the decision not to call for help, a decision which undoubtedly hastens her death. A theme running through the monologue is the fear Doris has of having to go into a nursing home. Eventually, her choice of risking dying alone was preferable to living in a nursing home. She reflects about that possibility:

> Mix, I don't want to mix. Comes to the finish and they suddenly think you want to mix. I don't want to be stuck with a lot of old lasses. And they all smell of pee. And daft half of them banging tambourines. You go daft there, there's nowhere else for you to go but daft. Wearing somebody else's frock. They even mix up your teeth. . . .

The strong message communicated in this story is the primacy of individual autonomy: we ought to be able to make our own decisions in life – and in death. Yet an equally poignant message, complementing the autonomy argument, is related to the sorts of caring relationships Doris would or would not expect. Doris's choice of death alone in preference to a place in a nursing home is a significant statement regarding the sort of care being provided.

Whilst Bennett (1988) can be excused an element of theatrical licence, the questions he raises are very pertinent to the theme of this book. What indeed is our response to the choice of death as opposed to a place in a nursing home? Is it really such a rare occurrence or do we know people who have resolutely 'turned their faces to the wall' and willed a hasty death? Can we learn anything about our responsibility to care for others when we hear such stories?

We have begun this concluding chapter in such a way as to remind ourselves of the major theme running through this book. It would have been relatively straightforward to provide an outline of the main moral principles, how they are selected and applied in moral deliberation and to illustrate these with a few relevant case studies. Yet what we have attempted to do is introduce a further dimension into debates on nursing ethics and that dimension is caring. What is caring? How does it relate to nursing? What are the moral foundations of caring? Is caring a virtue? Is a good nurse a virtuous carer?

There are some people in nursing who do not think explorations in the concept of caring are useful at all. Caring, they argue, is much too universal a concept, everyone does it, there is neither intellectual rigour nor clear understanding attached to the concept, and all it does is confuse activities carried out by nurses, doctors, social workers and so on. Indeed they go so far as to argue that to expect strangers, in this case professionals, to care for people when they are in need is preposterous. Professionals provide a service but, in the common sense way we tend to use the word 'caring', we ought never to expect professionals to care. It is beyond their duty.

This is an important view point to consider, and particularly as we in this book have attempted to illustrate how caring, like truth-telling and confidentiality for example, is intimately bound up in the ethical deportment of nurses when forming therapeutic relationships or doing things with their patients.

It may be that, as a concept, caring has been ignored because it has traditionally been related to woman's work and has thus tended not to be treated with the same measure of intellectual respect as other related concepts such as compassion or sympathy. In Chapter Three we have attempted to outline some of the current thinking about caring, drawing attention to those elements in its nature which lend themselves to ethical deliberation. It is interesting to note also the historical development of the concept (as graphically described in Colliere's paper, 1982) from that of a well respected skill – comparable and often equivalent to healing – to a task linked with domestic service. Such internal tensions captured within the concept have not yet been resolved. Attempts at legitimizing the more theoretical dimensions of caring have been taken up by psychotherapeutic literature in particular by authors such as Mayeroff (1971), May (1977) and Rogers (1961). Here, caring was acknowledged as an important aspect of human experience by putting it into a psychotherapeutic context.

While this wave of interest in the psychotherapeutic nature of caring was developing, little recognition was given to the ethical nature of caring. Early literature on nursing had exhorted the nurse to be dutiful, obedient, compassionate and kind. Implicit in these exhortations was the idea that the nurse knew how to care. Yet recent detailed analyses of caring which emphasize the need of the carer to immerse themselves in the experience of the one being cared for paints a different picture altogether.

The level of contact and intimacy expected in caring relationships is perhaps what makes professionals and others shy away from them. Armchair philosophy is tolerable; even discussions about life and death issues, confidentiality, truth-telling, respecting other peoples' wishes are acceptable when there is a certain intellectual distance between the thinker and the doer. But as we have tried to illustrate in the book, practical ethics is about marrying the ability to deliberate and come to good decisions while continuing to be involved with other peoples' life events.

Consideration of the caring relationship puts a different perspective on ethical deliberation. It grounds the decision-making process firmly into a context; that is, it demands the consideration of a particular set of conditions within a specific relationship at a certain place and time. Caring contextualizes ethical deliberation in a way that focuses the mind of the decision maker upon certain ethical principles underlying the nature of the caring relationship. For example, several case studies throughout the book have emphasized the importance of really knowing the other person before one can be expected to make a good decision for them. This was summarized as the birthday present problem. Many of the ethical dilemmas occur when there is conflict between one person's view of what is best for another person and that person's own view of what is best for themselves. Running through the argument for understanding ethical dimensions of caring is the need for the carer to be totally familiar with the desires, wishes, frustrations, limitations of the other person. This is not seen as an optional extra but as an essential element of an authentic caring relationship. Thus, if we were to stipulate in any future discussion on ethical deliberation that the one trying to make a decision for the other person, e.g. not telling a patient the truth of their prognosis or deciding that a particular treatment is what they need, had to provide evidence of the nature of their caring relationship then it would certainly realign certain priorities in the decision-making process.

Of course we are not saying that forming authentic caring relationships with one's clients will always lead to better ethical decisions being made. But what we are attempting to express is the need to take this concept more seriously and to treat it with more respect. Can certain elements of the concept be viewed as moral principles? Thus, alongside such principles as beneficence, nonmaleficence, respect and justice, there might be caring. As a principle guiding moral deliberation, it will have an internal consistency which will help the deliberator come to a right decision. Or is caring more of a virtue? Rather than its being viewed as a principle, should we be exhorting people to be caring people? Just as we extol discretion, honesty, patience and fortitude, should we be urging our readers to nurture the virtue of caring. And would this be called compassion?

Remember that the principle of confidentiality required the virtue of discretion, truth-telling that of honesty. So are we beginning to consider the possibility that moral principles may have certain 'naturally occurring' virtues co-existing with them? It may be that naturally caring people choose to be nurses just as we would hope that those who have the virtue of justness or fairness would end up as judges. But we cannot expect virtues alone to guide moral decision-making. In Chapter Two we outlined the five steps of moral deliberation. First there is the appreciation of the situation – having the facts, combining the rational with the contextual, i.e. what our intellect tells us about the case and what our senses communicate to us about this particular set of circumstances. Then we go through the possible courses of action open to us. Our grasp of what these are is likely to be influenced and perhaps distorted by our prior knowledge of moral principles, our personal strengths and weaknesses, and it is quite likely that we shall overlook some possibilities. Thus, the more mature student nurse in the example at the beginning of section 3.2 spotted (and took) a possibility of action that the younger ones did not see. But sometimes the more experienced person will move too confidently to one possibility and fail to see an option that is visible to younger, fresher eyes. Reflection on similar experiences, discussions with colleagues, our reflections on our own and others' motives for highlighting certain options all go towards helping us to correct or compensate for deficiencies in our initial review of the possibilities. Having identified the range of practical options open to us we then must decide which of these is preferable. On one level we tease out the underlying principles that are relevant to the situation and the courses of action as we now understand them. Then we try to take account of the reasons those principles give us for acting in one way rather than another; we also try to consider the range of consequences – both desired and unexpected – of each course of action, counting good consequences as a reason for taking that action and bad consequences as a reason for not taking it. The case study in Chapter Four works through a student nurse's deliberations regarding her role in helping an elderly patient make an informal choice about treatment. This and other examples in the book illustrate the delicacy of the deliberation, the often equally compelling arguments for one course of action or another, and how in reality decisions are never that clear cut. The final step in the process is actually making the decision – selecting one of the practical possibilities.

How do we know that we have made the right decision? The correct reply is in a sense we can never really be certain that we have made the right decision but we can look for a measure of certainty by checking our decision against the following factors. For example, our final decision ought to meet the requirements of the principle or principles selected at stage 3. If we have committed ourselves to the notion of caring as a major issue of primary consideration then our decision has to conform to our best notion of caring. The decision must also assure us that it offers the best for the client within a context – a different set of circumstances or context might have required a very different solution to the same ethical issue. And finally one should not ignore the sense that one has of oneself when making such decisions. You ought to be left with the sense that you have done the sort of thing you wanted to do and have been the sort of person that you are. If you are a virtuous person so much the better!

What is most important to communicate about ethics and nursing and caring is that you have to do it, or them, to be able to understand the complexities of the decision-making process. It is relatively straightforward to present the arguments for and against such things as abortion, euthanasia, artificial insemination or measures of the quality of another person's life. But when these principles are put into the context of another person's life with all the confusion and incompleteness that accompanies our everyday existence, then knowing what is the best thing to do is a different matter. Traditionally, professional groups have had codes of conduct or ethical codes to guide them (see Appendix), but these devices have never been seen to take the place of situation-based ethical decision-making.

Thus, we are constantly thrown back to the position of having to know how to make good decisions in complicated situations where there seem to be conflicting arguments about what we should do. The conflict may mask itself in the guise of interprofessional squabbles as outlined in Chapter Five. We should not permit traditional professional boundaries to cover more fundamental moral principles such as that of autonomy or respect for persons. In the same way, the real elements of the problem may be masked by institutional routines which people are reluctant to alter. There seems to be on the surface a vast difference between the desire to ensure that certain patients are fully informed about their treatment, prognosis and such like while others are not given the opportunity to choose where they are going to sit, what they are going to wear or whether they have the option of going to the toilet when they feel the urge to go.

From an ethical point of view is there any real difference between the potential loss of autonomy in the above cases? Is there anything to be said under the principle of justice about the different experience of different groups of people within the health care system? Have any of these situations got anything to do with the concept of caring as elaborated in the text? Reminding ourselves of Doris's choice, would she have selected differently if she had an alternative perception of professional care? Did she have any right to expect anything else?

Another feature of books such as this is that they raise more questions than they answer. We do not apologise for this and hope that the journey that we have taken, influenced by our own personal experiences, will spur others on to exploring more fully some of the issues raised.

Codes of nursing ethics

In this book we have sought to offer suggested concepts and terminology which might be found useful in deliberation and discussion of ethical problems which nurses encounter. In this appendix we consider the position of codes of conduct which can be looked on as intended to give ethical guidance to members of the nursing profession.

It is a fact of life that a person's decisions cannot be taken by any other person. (If someone else takes a decision, it is not *my* decision. I cannot be held responsible for it.) One of the things morality is about is getting one's decisions right, so that the things one decides to do are the *right* things to do.

A PERSON'S MORAL PRINCIPLES

Most people have some moral principles. That is to say, a person normally makes moral judgements or has moral views about all kinds of issues, and these views or judgements are shaped and guided by certain general principles. To say that Henry has principles of thrift and truthfulness is to say that these principles are among the principles guiding and shaping Henry's particular views and judgements. A person may or may not be aware of what his or her own principles are. One might try to identify one's own principles by putting into words a general moral statement and then seeing if the particular judgements one makes about various situations will square with that general statement. If the general statement conflicts with the particular judgements, then the general statement is not after all one of one's principles.

GENERAL MORALITY

Let us take it, then, that in this sense each of us has some moral principles, even though we might not have any very clear idea of exactly what they are. Granted that we all have some principles or other, no doubt some of us have better principles than others. In our factual beliefs, all of us have things to learn, and with luck we do learn things as life goes on. It seems reasonable to assume that people's principles also are imperfect and that most of us are wrong in some of our moral convictions. Let us say that general morality consists of those principles that each of us would have if we had moral principles which were not mistaken. Then, in a sense, a person's moral principles are that person's guess about what general morality is. The fact that we may be unclear about what our own moral principles are means that we may be unclear about what our guess about general morality is.

WHAT A CODIFICATION OF GENERAL MORALITY WOULD LOOK LIKE

In Chapter Two we noted various kinds of consideration that can enter into moral deliberation. There are considerations of duty or obligation, of rights, of value, and of virtue, etc. Moral principles concern the duty or obligation part of morality; if we put moral principles into words, what we have are universal normative statements. If we were to put a person's moral principles into words it would be as a collection of universal statements or rules (e.g. at *all* times lying is wrong, *all* promises should be respected, *no* child should be systematically humiliated). The general morality of conduct, if it can be codified at all, is codifiable as a set of universal normative statements. So a codification of general morality will be a collection of universal normative statements; likewise a partial codification of general morality will be a set of universal normative statements, but will not be the whole story about right and wrong conduct. To attempt to say what general morality is, in whole or in part, one has to offer a collection of universal normative statements.

MORAL PRINCIPLES AND REASONS FOR ACTION

When a principle applies to a situation, there is a moral reason for the relevant person to take the action indicated by that principle. Where two principles apply to the same situation, there may be moral reason for the person to act in one way but also moral reason for the same person to act in the opposite way: however, one reason may be weightier than another and, in that case, the comparative weight of the reasons will pick out an action as morally required. A strong principle is one which produces weighty reasons for action in the situations to which it applies; a weak principle produces reasons for action that are easily outweighed by other moral reasons for action.

PROFESSIONAL MORALITY AS A SPECIAL PART OF GENERAL MORALITY

If a situation has morally relevant features, general morality applies to that situation; there is something that any person in that situation ought – according to general morality – to do (e.g. if someone is in severe distress with no one to help him and you can help him without serious sacrifice or inconvenience, then you ought to). Now, members of a profession are obviously likely to be in situations of certain kinds; namely, those kinds that it is the business of the profession to deal with. So the possibility suggests itself that professional morality is just general morality as applied to those situations. Professional morality makes demands on persons in certain sorts of situations; it would make the same demands on anyone who was in such situations, but members of the profession are in them much more often than other people are, and are in them in the normal course of their work rather than fortuitously. It is therefore important that professionals bear in mind what general morality has to say about such situations, or be able without notice to bring to mind what general morality has to say about such situations or to respond without undue delay in a way that is informed by the implications of general morality for such situations. The only thing that is special about professional morality, then, is that it concerns special kinds of situations – situations which a good professional will be prepared for, morally as in other ways, and which there is no reason for other people to be particularly prepared for. What professional morality says about those special situations is not special; it is the very same thing that general morality says about them.

PROFESSIONAL MORALITY AS DISTINCT FROM GENERAL MORALITY

There is another possible view of professional morality, that it requires things of the members of a profession which general morality would not require of lay persons. It is generally accepted that social roles are defined in part by norms, and these include moral norms (cf. Beauchamp and Childress, 1983, p. 10). Professional roles – including the role of nurses – have to do with the promotion of certain values; to put it at its most general, nursing is concerned with promoting the values of human well-being, and the minimizing of suffering in sickness, injury, etc. All professionals are specialists of some kind; in their capacity as specialists (teachers, nurses, lawyers, etc.), they are concerned not with all values but rather with some special set of values. In their capacity as specialists, they will thus have to be what in the case of a lay person would be disproportionately concerned with those values.

Moreover, in view of their special concern with certain values, we would be wrong to rule out in advance the possibility that they will be subject to moral rules or principles of conduct which lay persons would not be subject to; and we would be wrong to rule out in advance the possibility that moral principles guiding professionals will have relative strengths differing from the relative strengths which the same principles would have in the case of lay persons. This is quite in keeping with the thought that different roles have their characteristic virtues, so that what is a virtue in a soldier or a civil servant may not be a virtue in a parent or a priest. In view of these considerations, it would be unwise to assume that professional morality is just general morality applied to a special range of situations which especially concern the professionals. We shall avoid taking it for granted that what professional morality requires is just the same as what general morality would require. So we shall be prepared to countenance the possibility that what a professional ought to do and what anyone ought to do might be two different things. But professionals are persons too. So we cannot just rule out the possibility of a conflict between professional morality and general morality, where general morality requires a person to do one thing and professional morality requires the same person to do the opposite.

WHAT A CODE OF PROFESSIONAL ETHICS DOES

If a certain problem occurs again and again, it is sensible to have a routine procedure for dealing with the problem. Then, when someone is faced with the problem yet another time, they do not need to start deciding what to do but can simply carry out the procedure. It would be nice if it were possible to codify nursing ethics by identifying the recurrent ethical problems in nursing, developing routine solutions for these problems and making the solutions known to members of the profession, thus saving each nurse's having to find out for herself or himself what to do each time one of those problems arose. But this is not possible. Ethical problems in nursing do not, in the main, present themselves in an orderly standard form for which routine solutions would be adequate. A code of nursing ethics cannot be expected to take people's decisions for them.

The claim of nursing to professional status is related to the nonmechanical character of nursing decisions. The literature of recent years shows a sustained effort to build up and consolidate both nurses' own perception of themselves as professionals (and not menials) and the public's perception of nursing as a profession. Part of what this involves is its becoming accepted that nurses do not just carry out orders but know what is going on, have their own expertise, corpus of research based knowledge, and so on. Now if nurses are to be perceived as autonomous co-workers rather than just followers of instructions, then they have to be seen as competent to face up to and cope with moral aspects of their work rather than unquestioningly carrying out what some moral instruction book says.

So what does a code of ethics do? It tries to make explicit the morality of the profession. This does not mean that an ethical code is definitive of the profession's ethics. In formulating a code, a profession is not *laying down* what is right and wrong for members of the profession. Rather, the position is that even before there is a code there are things which it is right for members of the profession to do and there are things which it is wrong (or unprofessional) for them to do; and in drawing up the code the profession – or its code of ethics working party – tries to say what these are. It tries to sum them up. It was suggested before that a person's moral principles are that person's guess about what morality is (or what it requires of us). We can now say that a code of professional ethics is the profession's guess about what the morality of the profession is. This is borne out by the fact that codes of nursing ethics tend to get changed from time to time. The practice of reviewing and revising codes of ethics shows that the codes are not thought of as being themselves the standards of right and wrong but are rather seen as imperfect but improving expressions of those standards.

A code does not *define* the ethics or morality of the profession. Rather, it attempts to *sum up* the profession's ethics; and in this it is almost certain to be less than completely successful. Consequently, there will practically always be room for improvement. This is reflected in the fact that major codes of nursing ethics, notably the ANA Code for Nurses and the ICN's International Code of Nursing Ethics, get revised from time to time. The first edition of the UKCC's Code of Professional Conduct, 1983 was rapidly followed by a second edition.

CODES DO NOT SUPERSEDE THINKING

The fact that codes get revised gives a way of bringing out quite emphatically the point that a code cannot be the whole story about nursing ethics. Suppose a committee has the task of reviewing an existing code with a view to making recommendations about whether the code needs changing and what changes should be made. Then one thing the committee cannot be guided by in making its deliberations is the old code. The committee members may be guided by the *spirit* of the old code and may suggest a new form of words in the light of that; they may identify what the old code was *trying* to say and look for a better way of saying it. In this case it is looking beyond the form of words of the old code, and is not being guided by that form of words. And, quite apart from whether the old code says well what it was trying to say, the committee members may well need to consider whether what the old code was trying to say was the right thing to be trying to say. In that case, the committee will be reconsidering the underlying ideas of the old code. And in deliberating about this the committee clearly cannot be guided by the old code itself. But the committee will be guided in its deliberations by considerations belonging to the morality of the profession. So it is clear that the code cannot be the whole story about that morality.

Thus it cannot be the case that professional ethics codes make all moral thinking unnecessary for members of the profession. For the profession has to do at least such moral thinking as is involved in the periodic review of its ethics code. However, this still leaves open the possibility that, in between the periodic reviews of an ethics code, the code obviates the need for moral thinking. But this is not the case either.

As was noted above, the possibility cannot be ruled out that general morality and professional morality will conflict in particular instances. If this is correct then, even where a code is a perfect expression of professional ethics, the code might in some particular cases be in conflict with general morality. If such a case were actually to arise, a nurse – as a responsible moral agent – would have to consider whether to follow general morality or professional ethics. In other words, the nurse would have to do some moral thinking. Now, since it *might* be that such cases will arise, what nurses can't properly do is go onto automatic pilot and simply disconnect their capacity for moral thinking except at such times as they might be called upon to serve on committees reviewing their ethics code.

DESIDERATA AND LIMITATIONS

There is another kind of reason why the need for moral thinking is not obviated in the intervals between code reviews. The primary purpose of an ethics code, as Muyskens (1982, pp. 7–8) puts it, 'is to provide a concise statement of the principles that should guide a nurse's actions'. So an ethics code has to be concise or brief. It also has to be such as to have the general assent of the profession. Both of these considerations point towards a code's being to some extent vague and general. And this means that there will be many cases on which the code will not yield clear and unequivocal guidance. (Benjamin and Curtis (1981, p. 8) offer a variant of the same argument. They point out that a brief, simple code might gain widespread acceptance but will not give clear guidance, and that a long, detailed code might offer clear guidance but will not command widespread acceptance. Consequently, no code can both give clear guidance and attain widespread acceptance.)

There are various things that we might ask of a code of ethics. For a start, it should be understandable. Further, it should be easy to commit to memory. In addition, it should be comprehensive; i.e., it should be the whole story about right and wrong for the profession. And it should be specific, so that the story is not left vague but includes all the details. Finally, it should be acceptable. Now, as Benjamin and Curtis (1981) argue, it is inevitable that a code of professional ethics will be imperfect in the sense that it cannot possibly satisfy all these desiderata. In particular, in a pluralist society, you can be confident that the more specific a code gets on some issues, the more unlikely it is to command the universal assent of the members of the profession. So any code of nursing ethics will have to be a compromise between the various desiderata. It will have inherent limitations.

The inherent, unavoidable limitations of ethics codes do not mean, though, that ethics codes give no guidance at all. On the contrary, a code that is brief and simple but well thought out will give clear and unequivocal guidance for very many of the situations that nurses are likely to encounter in the ordinary way of things. The point of the foregoing is not that nurses need to be constantly agonizing about whether their professional code will keep them right or not; the point is rather that as a responsible moral agent the nurse has to be ready to cope with cases where, even in the light of the code, it is not immediately clear what is morally required.

Muyskens (1982, p. 11) observes that the ICN and ANA codes 'set the boundaries and outline the ideals for proper nursing practice'. He summarizes their position thus: 'the professional codes provide an excellent starting-point from which to launch a systematic investigation of the moral problems of nursing. But because of their brevity, vagueness, generality, and incompleteness, they are not an appropriate end-point.'

SHARED BACKGROUND

We have suggested that a professional code is a profession's guess at what its ethics is; it represents the profession's most recent – and perhaps best yet – attempt to articulate briefly its ethics. Despite the inevitable limitations of any such code, it will give some guidance as to how to act. It will also have practical relevance in another way. It will serve an agenda-setting function for anyone engaged in deliberation or discussion about an ethical issue; by highlighting certain themes, it will in effect invite nurses to give a central place in their discussion or deliberation to those themes.

It will also facilitate discussion by being something to which any individual can refer in the confident knowledge that others will grasp the reference. It will articulate a body of shared assumptions common to members of the profession – or at least assumptions concerning which everyone will know that they are expected to be shared. If a nurse in discussion with colleagues makes reference to taking account of patients' customs and values, she can be confident that her colleagues will view that as a consideration not to be dismissed out of hand. If she introduces into discussion some idea not incorporated in a code or otherwise current, she will know that she may have to reckon with having to explain what the idea is about. So a professional code assists people in discussions by letting them know what they can take for granted and what they might have to explain from the ground up.

A special case of such discussion is the case where a junior nurse feels that standards of care have slipped to an unacceptable level and is trying to get others to agree that improvement is needed. Having the profession's code to appeal to can be of immeasurable help. It gives her the assurance that her feelings are not something peculiar or eccentric and that she is not alone in having the concerns she has, and that if others do not see what she is talking about then they ought to.

According to UKCC registrar Colin Ralph, many nurses, midwives and health visitors, particularly clinical staff, look to the UKCC code of conduct as a guide to ethical issues. 'We know that many junior staff, struggling to maintain standards of care for their patients, draw strength from the code in bringing attention to deficiencies,' he says.

(Pownall, 1989)

At the same time, the ideas expressed in a code can prompt development in discussion by having implications which are not determinate or specifiable in advance. Exactly what taking account of customs and values is to involve in practice is something that nurses can develop in consideration of concrete situations. A code can aid the development and growth of the profession's ethics by presenting leading ideas which invite discussion and can be worked out in it.

It was suggested in Chapter One that criticism of ideas and conjectures is an important part of enquiry. The continuing development of a profession's understanding of itself and its ethics is a form of enquiry. By articulating the profession's current understanding of its ethics, a code facilitates criticism of that understanding; and through criticism comes improvement. Having a printed, published code of conduct enables a profession to sharpen up its understanding of its ethics through critical appraisal of the code.

Although not describing itself as an ethical code, the UKCC Code fulfils this function and is accompanied by a notice stressing the profession's responsibility to keep the code itself under continuous review.

CHANGING CODES

Inspection of the ICN Code for Nurses of 1953 and 1965 and that of 1973 shows a marked shift in the way the profession is conceived. There is of course no suggestion that, in medical matters, the nurse ceases to be a recipient and implementer of doctors' instructions. But that aspect of nursing practice no longer seems to be regarded as setting the tone for nursing practice in general. Instead, what emerges from the 1973 code is that the nurse is more co-worker than servant and often has to exercise judgement in a mature and informed way (cf. RCN Code of Professional Conduct – A Discussion Document IV(1) . . . 'free discussion of the reasons for established procedures should be encouraged at all levels.' Tate, 1977, p. 98). Moreover the right of a nurse to a private life of his/ her own choosing is tacitly acknowledged. (This is explicit in the RCN's discussion document, section V, in Tate, 1977, p. 100.)

Also, the 1953 and 1965 stark assertion of a fundamental responsibility to conserve life is weakened; instead of that fundamental responsibility we have this: 'Inherent in nursing is respect for life, dignity and rights of man.' Thus there is no longer anything that could be construed as an injunction to conserve life at all costs (cf. the RCN document, discussion to II(4): 'For instance a nurse may question whether the dignity of a dying patient is being respected by procedures employed to delay death.' Tate, 1977, p. 97.)

Whereas item 4 of the 1965 International Code of Nursing Ethics says simply that nurses are to hold in confidence personal information entrusted to them, the 1973 version adds that they are to use judgement in sharing such information. Whereas item 9 of the 1965 Code affirms nurses' entitlement to just remuneration, the 1973 Code is much clearer and presents nurses as active in securing equitable working conditions rather than only as having an entitlement.

Change is not necessarily in the direction of greater specificity. The 1965 Code, item 7, affirms 'an obligation to carry out the physician's orders intelligently and loyally and to refuse to participate in unethical procedures'. The 1973 Code says 'the nurse takes appropriate action to safeguard the individual when his care is endangered by a co-worker or any other person'. This is not only less authoritarian but also more vague than the earlier version. Thus the nurse is more a co-worker and less a servant, and the nurse is to exercise judgement about what to do and not just implement a prescribed procedure; also she or he has to exercise judgement about what is an instance of care being endangered.

Both the introduction to the 1976 ANA Code for Nurses ('it is imposs-ible to anticipate in a code every type of situation that may be encountered in professional practice') and the RCN Discussion Document ('no code can do justice to every individual case') acknowledge that no code will be the whole story about ethically correct professional conduct. The RCN document goes on to stress the importance of sustained discussion among nurses and others.

Thus the tendency is away from unthinking acceptance of actual prac-tices and towards critical and reflective consideration of those practices.

References

Anscombe, G. E. M. (1981) *Ethics, Religion and Politics*, Basil Blackwell, Oxford.

Aquinas, St Thomas (1265–1273) Whether it is lawful to kill oneself, in *Summa Theologica*, reprinted in Beauchamp, Tom L. and Perlin, S. (1978) (eds), *Ethical Issues in Death and Dying*, Prentice-Hall, Englewood Cliffs, New Jersey, 102–05.

Beauchamp, Tom L. and Childress, James F. (1983) *Principles of Biomedical Ethics*, 2d edn., Oxford University Press, Oxford.

Beauchamp, Tom L. and McCullough, L. (1984) *Medical Ethics, the Moral Responsibility of Physicians*, Prentice-Hall, Englewood Cliffs, New Jersey.

Beauchamp, Tom L. and Perlin, S. Date (1978), (eds) *Ethical Issues in Death and Dying*, Prentice-Hall, Englewood Cliffs, New Jersey.

Bell, J. M. and Mendus, Susan (1988) (eds) *Philosophy and Medical Welfare*, Cambridge University Press, Cambridge.

Benjamin, M. and Curtis, J. (1981) *Ethics in Nursing*, Oxford University Press, New York.

Benn, S. I. (1984) Privacy, freedom, and respect for persons, in Schoeman, F. P. (1984) (ed.), *Philosophical Dimensions of Privacy*, Cambridge University Press, Cambridge, 223–44.

Bennet, A. (1988) A cream cracker under the settee, in, *Talking Heads*, BBC Books, London.

Blackham, H. J. (1959) *Six Existentialist Thinkers*, Routledge and Kegan Paul, London.

Bok, S. (1980) *Lying*, Quartet Books, London.

Bok, S. (1984) *Secrets*, Oxford University Press, Oxford.

Bosk, C. L. (1979) *Forgive and Remember: Managing Medical Failure*, University of Chicago Press, Chicago, Illinois.

Brewer, C. (1988) Should Doctors control discharge? *Nursing Times*, **84**, (3), 42.

Broome, John (1984) The Economic Value of Life, *Economics*, **52**, 281–294.

Broome, John Notes on QALYs. *Ian Ramsey Centre Report*, **2**, Banner, Michael and Mitchel, Basil (eds), Basil Blackwell, Oxford.

Broome, John (1988) Good, fairness and QALYs, in Bell, J. M. and Mendus, Susan (1988) (eds), *Philosophy and Medical Welfare*, Cambridge University Press, Cambridge.

Broome, John (1990) Fairness. *Proceedings of the Aristotelian Society*, **XCI**, 1990/91, 87–102.

Brown, S., Fauvel, J. and Finnegan, R. (1981), *Conceptions of Inquiry*, Methuen, London.

Buber, M. (1958) *I and Thou*, Ronald Gregor Smith (trans.), reprinted 1984, T & T Clark Ltd, Edinburgh.

Campbell, A. V. (1984a) *Moderated Love*, SPCK, London.

Campbell, A. V. (1984b) *Moral Dilemmas in Medicine*, Churchill Livingstone, Edinburgh.

Canadian Nurses Association (1980) *CNA Code of ethics*, Canadian Nurses Association, Ottawa, Canada.

Clark, Justice William P. (1981) Dissenting opinion, in *Tarasoff v. Regents of the University of California*, in Mappes, Thomas A. and Zembaty, Jane S. (1981) (eds), *Biomedical Ethics*, McGraw-Hill, 124–7.

Colliere, M. F. (1986) Invisible care and invisible women as health care providers. *International Journal of Nursing Studies*, **23** (2), 95–112.

Collins, J. (1981) Should doctors tell the truth?, in Mappes, Thomas A. and Zembaty, Jane S. (1981) (eds), *Biomedical Ethics*, McGraw-Hill, 64–7.

Curtin, Leah and Flaherty, M. Josephine (1982) *Nursing Ethics*, Brady, Bowie, Maryland.

Davis, A. J. and Aroskar, M. A. (1978) *Ethical Dilemmas and Nursing Practice*, Appleton-Century-Crofts, New York.

Dennett, Daniel C. (1982) Mechanism and responsibility, in Watson, Gary (1982) (ed.), *Free Will*, Oxford University Press, Oxford, 150–73.

Dock, S. (1917) The relation of the nurse to the doctor and the doctor to the nurse. *American Journal of Nursing*, **17**, 394.

Downie, R. S. and Calman, K. C. (1987) *Healthy Respect*, Faber and Faber, London.

Dworkin, R. M. (ed.) (1977) *The Philosophy of Law*, Oxford University Press, Oxford.

Edelstein, L (1943) Oath of Hippocrates, in *The Hippocratic Oath: Text, Translation and Interpretation. Bulletin of the History of Medicine*, supplement 1, Johns Hopkins University Press, Baltimore, Maryland.

English, Jane (1987) Abortion and the concept of a person, in Mappes, Thomas A. and Zembaty, Jane S. (1987) (eds), *Social Ethics*, 3d edn, McGraw-Hill, New York, 29–38.

Evans, John Grimley (1987) The sanctity of life, in *Medical Ethics and Elderly People*, Elford, John (ed.), Churchill Livingstone, Edinburgh.

Fairbairn, G. and Fairbairn, S. (1988) (eds) *Ethical Issues in Caring*, Avebury, Aldershot.

Fitzpatrick, P. (1984) Lay concepts of illness, in Fitzpatrick, R., Hinton, J., Newman, S., Scampbler, G., Thompson, J., *The Experience of Illness* (1984), Tavistock Publications, London.

Fradd, J. (1988) Tug of love. *Nursing Times*, **84** (41), 32–5.

Fried, C. (1984) Privacy, in Schoeman, F. D. (1984) (ed.), *Philosophical Dimensions of Privacy*, Cambridge University Press, Cambridge, 203–22.

Gerstein, R. S. (1984) Intimacy and privacy, in Schoeman, F. D. (1984) (ed.), *Philosophical Dimensions of Privacy*, Cambridge University Press, Cambridge, 265–71.

Gilligan, C. (1982) *In a Different Voice*, Harvard University Press, Cambridge, Mass., USA.

Gillon, R. (1986) *Philosophical Medical Ethics*, John Wiley, Chichester.

Gillon, R. (1989) Editorial – Funding and efficiency in the National Health Service. *Journal of Medical Ethics*, **15**, 115–16, 128.

Glover, J. (1977) *Causing Death and Saving Lives*, Penguin, Harmondsworth.

Glover, J. (1984) *What Sort of People Should There Be?*, Penguin, Harmondsworth.

Glover, J. *et al.* (1989) *Fertility & the Family*, Fourth Estate, London.

Goldman, H. S. (1980) Killing, letting die, and euthanasia. *Analysis*, **40** (4), 224.

Gregory, J. (1817) *Lectures on the Duties and Qualifications of a Physician*, M. Carey & Son, Philadelphia.

Griffin, A. P. (1983) A philosophical analysis of caring in nursing. *Journal of Advanced Nursing*, **8**, 289–95.

Griffin, A. P. (1980) Philosophy and nursing. *Journal of Advanced Nursing*, **5**, 261–72.

Gustafson, J. (1973) Mongolism, parental desires and the right to life. *Perspectives in Biology and Medicine*, **16**, 555.

Harman, G. (1977) *The Nature of Morality*, Oxford University Press, New York.

Harris, John (1985) *The Value of Life*, Routledge and Kegan Paul, London.

Harris, J. (1987) QALYfying the value of life. *Journal of Medical Ethics*, **13** (3), September, 117–23.

Harris, John (1988a) EQALYty, in *King's College Studies*, Peter Byrne (ed.), King's Fund, London.

Harris, John (1988b) More and better justice, in Bell, J. M. and Mendus, Susan (1988) (eds), *Philosophy and Medical Welfare*, Cambridge University Press, Cambridge.

Heidegger, M. (1962) *Being and Time*, Blackwell, Oxford.

Henderson, V. (1966) *The Nature of Nursing*, Collier Macmillan, West Drayton.

Hilfiker, D. (1985) *Healing the Wounds*, Pantheon, New York.

Holland, A. (1984) On behalf of moderate speciesism. *Journal of Applied Philosophy*, **1** (2), 281–91.

Holland, A. (1990) A fortnight of my life is missing. *Journal of Applied Philosophy*, **7** (1), 25–37.

Hume, D. (1777) On Suicide. Page references to reprint in Beauchamp, Tom L. and Perlin, S. (1978) (eds), *Ethical Issues in Death and Dying*, Prentice-Hall, Englewood Cliffs, New Jersey, 105–10.

Hursthouse, R. (1987) *Beginning Lives*, Basil Blackwell, Oxford.

Institute of Medical Ethics Working Party (1990) Assisted death. *The Lancet*, **336** (8715), September 8, 610–13.

International Council of Nurses (1973) *ICN Code for Nurses – Ethical Concepts Applied to Nursing*, International Council of Nurses, Geneva.

International Council of Nurses (1986) *Report on the Regulation of Nursing*, Geneva.

Kant, I. (1785) *Groundwork of the Metaphysics of Morals*, (Various editions and translations available).

Kind, P., Rosser, R. and Williams A. (1982) Valuation of quality of life, in *The Value of Life and Safety*, Jones-Lee MW (ed.), Elsevier/North-Holland, Amsterdam.

Kitson, Alison (1987) A comparative analysis of lay caring and professional (nursing) care relationships. *International Journal of Nursing Studies*, **24** (2), 155–165.

Kitson, Alison, (1988) On the concept of nursing care, in Fairburn, G. and Fairburn S. (1988) (eds), *Ethical Issues in Caring*, Avebury, Aldershot, 21–31.

Komrad, M. (1983) A defence of medical paternalism: maximising patents' autonomy. *Journal of Medical Ethics*, **9**, 38–44.

Kuhse, H. (1987) *The Sanctity-of-Life Doctrine in Medicine*, Clarendon Press, Oxford.

Kuhse, H. and Singer, P. (1985) *Should the Baby Live?*, Oxford University Press, Oxford.

Lamb (1981) Nursing Ethics in Canada: Two Decades. Unpublished Master's Thesis, University of Alberta, Edmonton, Alberta.

Linacre Centre Working Party (1982) *Euthansia and Clinical Practice*, The Linacre Centre, London.

Lockwood, M. (1988) Quality of life and resource allocation, in Bell, J. M. and Mendus, Susan (1978) (eds), *Ethical Issues in Death and Dying*, Prentice-Hall, Englewood Cliffs, New Jersey.

Loomes, G. and McKenzie, L. (1989) The use of QALYs in health care decision making. *Society of Scientific Medicine*, **28** (4), 299–308.

MacIntyre, Alasdair (1981) *After Virtue*, Gerald Duckworth, London.

Magee, Bryan (1973) *Popper*, London: Fontana/Collins.

Mappes, Thomas A. and Zembaty, Jane S. (1981) (eds), *Biomedical Ethics*, McGraw-Hill, New York.

Mappes, Thomas A. and Zembaty, Jane S. (1987) (eds) *Social Ethics*, 3d edn, McGraw-Hill, New York.

Marshall, S. E. (1988) Public bodies, private selves. *Journal of Applied Philosophy*, **5** (2), 147–58.

Maslow, A. H. (1954) *Motivation and Personality*, Harper & Row, New York.

May, W. F. (1975) Code, covenant, contract, or philanthropy. *The Hastings Center Report* **5** (6), 37.

May, W. F. (1977) Code and covenant or philanthropy and contract?, in Reiger, S. J., Dyck, A. J. and Curran, W. J. (eds), *Ethics in Medicine*, MIT Press, Cambridge, Massachusetts.

Mayeroff, Milton (1971) *On Caring*, Harper & Row, New York.

McCulloch, Douglas (1989) *Who Needs QALYs?*. Policy Planning and Research Unit. Occasional Paper No. 19, Economics Division, Policy Planning and Research Unit.

McCulloch, Douglas (1990) The development of the QALY approach – A research project. Unpublished manuscript, copies available from author, Department of Applied Economics and Human Resource Management, University of Ulster at Jordanstown.

McDowell, John (1979) Virtue and reason. *The Monist*, **62** (3), 331–50.

McFarlane, J. (1988) Nursing: a paradigm of caring, in Fairburn, G. and Fairburn, S. (1988) (eds), *Ethical Issues in Caring*, Avebury, Aldershot, 10–20.

McNeil, B. J., Weichselbaum, R. and Pauker, S. G. (1981) Speech and survival: Tradeoffs between quality and quantity of life in laryngeal cancer. *New England Journal of Medicine*, **305**, 982–7.

Meisel, A. and Roth, L. H. (1981) What we do and do not know about informed consent. *Journal of the American Medical Association* **246**, 27 November, 2473–7.

Melia, Kath (1983) Becoming and being a nurse, in Thompson, *et al.*, (1983) *Nursing Ethics*, Churchill Livingstone, Edinburgh.

Menzies, I. E. P. (1970) *The Functioning of Social Systems as a Defence Against Anxiety*, Tavistock, London.

Midgley, M. (1980) *Beast and Man*, Methuen, London.

Mooney, G. H. (1986) *Economics, Medicine and Health Care* Harvester Wheat-sheaf, London.

Mooney, G. H. (1989) QALYs: are they enough? A health economist's perspective. *Journal of Medical Ethics*, **15**, 148–52.

Moore, T. V. (1935) *Principles of Ethics*, 4th edn, J. B. Lippincott, Philadelphia, Pennsylvania.

Muyskens, J. L. (1982) *Moral Problems in Nursing*, Rowman and Littlefield, Totowa, New Jersey.

Nagel, Thomas (1986) *The View from Nowhere*, Oxford University Press, Oxford.

Noddings, Nel (1984) *Caring*, University of California Press, Berkeley, California.

Nozick, R. (1988) Side constraints, in Scheffler, S. (1988) (ed.), *Consequentialism and its Critics*, Oxford University Press, Oxford, 134–41.

O'Neill, O. (1984a) How can we individuate a moral problem?, in Attig. T., *et al.* (eds), *Social Policy and Conflict Resolution*, The Applied Philosophy Program, Bowling Green, Ohio.

O'Neill, O. (1984b) Paternalism and partial autonomy, *Journal of Medical Ethics*, **10** 173–8.

Orem, D. (1980) *Nursing: Concepts of Practice*, 2d ed., McGraw-Hill, New York.

Orlando, I. J. (1961) *The Dynamic Nurse-Patient Relationship* New York, G. P. Putnam's Sons, New York.

Osler, W. (1904) *Aequanimities in Aequanimitas: With other Addresses to Medical Students, Nurses and Practitioners of Medicine*, Blakiston's Son & Company, Philadelphia, Pennsylvania.

Overall, C. (1985), New reproductive technology. *Journal of Value Inquiry*, **19** 279–92.

Parkes, C. M. (1975) *Bereavement*, Penguin Books, Harmondsworth.

Pearce, E. (1969) *Nurse and Patient*, 3d edn., Faber and Faber, London.

Pellegrino, E. (1979) Towards a reconstruction of medical morality: The primacy of the act of profession and the fact of illness. *Journal of Medicine and Philosophy*, **4** 32–46.

Percival, T. (1975) *Percival's Medical Ethics*, Chauncey Leake (ed.), Robert Krieger Publishing Company, Huntingdon, New York. (Reprint of Percival's *Medical Ethics* (1803) S. Russell, Manchester, England.)

Phillips, M. and Dawson, J. (1985) *Doctors' Dilemmas*, Harvester Press, Brighton.

Popper, K. R. (1969) *Conjectures and Refutations*, 3d edn, Routledge and Kegan Paul, London.

Pownall, M. (1989) When care has to be rationed. *Nursing Times*, **85** (5).

Rachels, J. (1986) *The end of life*, Oxford University Press, Oxford.

Rawles, J. (1989) Castigating QALYs. *Journal of Medical Ethics*, **15**, 143–7.

Rhodes, M. L. (1986) *Ethical Dilemmas in Social Work Practice*, Routledge and Kegan Paul, London.

Richards, Tessa and Beecham, Linda (1986) The BMA in Oxford. *British Medical Journal*, **292** (26), 1119–20.

Roach, M. S. (1984) *Caring, the Human Mode of Being, Implications for Nursing*, University of Toronto, Toronto, Ontario.

Rogers, C. (1961) *On Becoming a Person*, Houghton Mifflin, Boston, Massachusetts.

Ross, S. C. (1982) Abortion and the death of the fetus. *Philosophy and Public Affairs*, **11**, 232–45.

Royal College of Nursing (1980) *Guidelines on Confidentiality in Nursing*, Royal College of Nursing, London.

Royal College of Nursing (1986) *What the RCN stands for*, Royal College of Nursing, London.

Royal College of Nursing (1987) *In Pursuit of Excellence: A Position Statement on Nursing*, Royal College of Nursing London.

Ryden M. (1978) An approach to ethical decision-making. *Nursing Outlook*, November, 706–7.

Sainsbury, E. (1974) *Social Work with Families*, London, Routledge and Kegan Paul, London.

Salvage, Jane (1985) *The Politics of Nursing*, William Heinemann, London.

Saunders, C. *et al.* (1981) (eds) *Hospice: the living idea*, Edward Arnold, London.

Saunders, C. and Baines, M. (1989) *Living with Dying*, Oxford University Press, Oxford.

Schoeman, F. D. (1984) (ed) *Philosophical Dimensions of Privacy*, Cambridge University Press, Cambridge.

Schröck, R. A. (1980) A question of honesty in nursing practice. *Journal of Advanced Nursing*, **5**, 135–48.

Shelly, Judith Allen (1980) *Dilemma*, Inter Varsity Press, Downers Grove, Illinois.

Siegler, M. (1977) Critical illness: The limits of autonomy. *The Hastings Center Report*, 7 October, 12–15.

Singer, P. (1979) *Practical Ethics*, Cambridge University Press, Cambridge.

Singer, P. and Wells, D. (1984) *The Reproduction Revolution*, Oxford University Press, Oxford.

Smart, J. J. C. and Williams, Bernard (1973) *Utilitarianism – For and Against*, Cambridge University Press, Cambridge.

Sontag, S. (1978) *Illness as Metaphor*, Penguin, Harmondsworth.

Stinson, S. M. (1979) Nursing Research: The state of the art, in *Proceedings of the Kellogg International Seminar on Doctoral Preparation for Canadian Nurses*, Glennis Silm *et al.* (eds), Canadian Nurses' Association, Ottawa, Ontario.

Stinson, G. V. and Webb, B. (1975) *Going to See the Doctor: The Consultations Process in General Practice*, Routledge and Kegan Paul, London.

Strawson, Sir Peter (1982) Freedom and resentment, in Watson, Gary (ed.), *Free Will*, Oxford University Press, Oxford 59–80.

Szasz, T. and Hollender, M. (1956) A contribution to the philosophy of medicine: Three basic models of the doctor-patient relationship. *Archives of Internal Medicine* **97**, 585–92.

Tate, B. L. (1977) *The Nurse's Dilemma*, International Council of Nurses, Geneva.

Taylor, S. B., Pickens, J. and Geden, E. (1989) International styles of nurse practitioners and physicians regarding patient decision making. *Nursing Research*, **38**, 50–5.

Thompson, Ian E., Melia, Kath M. and Boyd, Kenneth M. (1983) *Nursing Ethics*, Churchill Livingstone, Edinburgh.

Thomson, J. J. (1977) A defence of abortion, in Dworkin, R. M. (1977) (ed.), *The Philosophy of Law*, Oxford University Press, Oxford, 112–28.

Tobriner, Justice Matthew O. (1981) Majority opinion, in *Tarasoff v. Regents of the University of California*, in Mappes, Thomas A. and Zembaty Jane S. (1981) (eds), *Biomedical Ethics*, McGraw-Hill, New York, 119–23.

Travelbee, J. (1971) *Interpersonal Aspects of Nursing*, 2d edn, Philadelphia, F. A. Davis, Philadelphia, Pennsylvania.

UKCC (1984) *Code of Professional Conduct for the Nurse, Midwife and Health Visitor*, 2nd edn., London.

UKCC (1987) *Confidentiality*, A UKCC Advisory Paper, London.

Veatch, R. (1981) *A Theory of Medical Ethics*, Basic Books, New York.

Walters, Leroy (1981) The principle of medical confidentiality, in Mappes, Thomas A. and Zembaty, Jane S. (1981) (eds), *Biomedical Ethics*, McGraw-Hill, New York, 116–19.

Walters, W. and Singer, P. (1982) *Test-Tube Babies*, Oxford University Press, Oxford.

Warnock, Dame Mary (1984) *Report of the Committee of Inquiry into Human Fertilisation and Embryology*, HMSO, London.

Warren, Mary Anne (1987) On the moral and legal status of abortion, in Mappes, Thomas A. and Zembaty, Jane S. (1987) (eds), *Social Ethics*, McGraw-Hill, New York, 14–21.

Wiggins, David (1978) Deliberation and practical reason in Raz, Joseph (1978) (ed.), *Practical Reasoning*, University Press, Oxford, 144–52.

Williams, Alan (1985a) The Value of QALYs. *Health and Social Service Journal*, 18 July, Centre 8, 3–5.

Williams, Alan (1985b) Economics of coronary artery bypass grafting. *British Medical Journal*, **291**, 3 August, 326–9.

Wittgenstein, L. (1961) *Tractatus Logico-Philosophicus*, Routledge and Kegan Paul, London.

Yarling, R. R. and McElmurry, B. J. (1986) The Moral Foundations of Nursing. *Advances in Nursing Science*, **8** (2), 63–73.

Index